T0105985

THIRTEEN TUNNELS

SUZANNE SAMPLES

RUNNING
Wild
PRESS

for Jeramy & the Mothman

Now this is the truth if I ever told it. This is not just a story.
—Mayme Samples Cole, my paternal great aunt whom I never met, but according to my Uncle Mack, was a "great ghost storyteller" and "a good shot with a pistol"[1]

The report of my death was an exaggeration.
—Mark Twain, but not really

I'm going back to that Swannanoa Tunnel,
That's my home, baby, that's my home.
Asheville Junction, Swannanoa Tunnel,
All caved in, baby, all caved in.
"Swannanoa Tunnel" (variation of "Nine Pound Hammer"),
English Folk Songs from the Southern Appalachians, collected by Cecil Sharp

THE BEFORE

I need to confess: The last four years have been a lie I didn't know I was telling.

West Union, West Virginia, Central Station Tunnel, #6, 2297 ft.

Upon discovering they have a terminal illness, some people have vacations on their bucket list.

I have thirteen tunnels.

I didn't plan for this, but when my mom announced I was moving home, I needed something to occupy my time. With some creative research involving a lot of oral history, I discovered there were thirteen abandoned train tunnels either on or near the North Bend Rail Trail, and all of the unlucky number were within a short driving distance of my town.

The Central Station Tunnel, #6, is the longest and most well-preserved tunnel I've encountered. I feel like an actual urban explorer (a faraway goal of mine since my disability prevents me from climbing into abandoned, haunted hospitals and churches, which would be the ultimate dream) as I enter the passageway. Though I'm alone and see no one else, whispers scatter like mice when I'm deep in the vestibule and shrouded from daylight. Slightly claustrophobic, I'm able to explore these structures without problem because although the light quickly disintegrates, plenty of space still provides breathing room.

It's time I'm unsure about.

Just like my sense of hours and minutes after brain surgery, seconds disappear in these tunnels.

A quick fog in the night.

I walk in at 1:15 p.m., and though most are only a few hundred feet, I might find myself in a tunnel for over an hour.

My parents are concerned, but like everything else they might need to worry about, they just pretend it's not happening.

Tunnel #6, as I feel with my feet, seems to have gritty sand on the bottom. The walls, from what I can see with my headlamp, look scrubbed clean like a white hospital. This is in clear contrast to the other eight tunnels I've seen so far, which, marred by time, water, and the ghosts of train conductors past, look like they might cave in at any moment. This tunnel, if it had a track, could still be in use.

I hope I didn't miss a track somewhere, or I might be in trouble.

Shadows, my own and others, dance past soundlessly, but I am not scared. What's in my body frightens me way more than anything in this tunnel.

In most of these passageways, you can see a keyhole of light at the other end, but this one is so long, it's just a ten-and-a-half-minute hallway of darkness. This tunnel, however, does not feel haunted; some have a heaviness you can feel as soon as you enter. It's hard to discern if this ponderous, solemn feeling comes from the 1800s or more modern monstrosities of contemporary times (how many women have been assaulted in these dark, private areas?), but some tunnels have a palpable residual energy that grips onto your headlamp and stays long after you exit into the light.

Tunnel #6 is completely chill and modern, though.

Dark but chill.

You know.

I feel like I'm shuffling through a dream where I'm in a deep sleep, but absolutely nothing is happening.

I am resting.

I feel protected.

I am nowhere.

I decide to hang out in the tunnel for a bit; sometimes I pass straight through them, take a couple pics, then get home, but this one seems free from negative energy and potential human threats. I charged my headlamp on my parents' new couch (technology! charging a headlamp on a couch!), and I have nothing else to do today.

I woke up early with a mission to find the North Bend Rail Trail's longest tunnel, and though the hike up the mountain nearly destroyed me, I made it.

West Union, West Virginia, away from the Central Station Tunnel, #6, 2297 ft.

On my way back from Tunnel #6, The Mothman flies above my busted jaw to welcome me home.

Originally reported as a "Man-Sized Bird ... Creature ... Something,[1]" The Mothman has haunted the hills of West Virginia since the mid-60s and is rumored to be responsible for the collapse of the Point Pleasant Silver Bridge in 1967 and scaring the shit out of Appalachians[2] for decades thereafter. A giant winged, black creature with glowing red eyes, some believe the West Virginia Mothman to be an alien; some see him as a mythical cryptid; some of the more logical hill folk

5

think he's simply a rather enormous, barred owl with a legendary fan base; some know him as a movie monster hotly pursued by Richard Gere, whose Chapstick can now be viewed in the Point Pleasant Mothman Museum for the small fee of $8.

Dearest Mothman, I call from the ground. I need your help. The world's gone to shit, and if Jesus can't save us, only you might be able to; call your old friend Indrid Cold[3] and have him gear up his spaceship to come and get us, me at the very least.

I don't know if I can get up this time. I fell on my way back from Tunnel #6, and I am only able to reach one of my hiking poles. I don't think the aluminum is strong enough to lift me; even if I can use the pole to get myself up, looking down at the steep rocky hillside does not give me faith I will safely reach the bottom—or reach the bottom at all.

Gazing up at the blue West Virginia sky, I realize I am fucked.

So fucked.

If I don't have a broken jaw, I might have a concussion; however, it's West Virginia, and it's Covid, so this does not matter. These are minor injuries I will not risk my life for, if, in fact, I do make it off this rockslide. I try to imagine EMTs potentially getting a stretcher up here; I'm not far from the road, and I can hear and almost see cars whooshing by. Strong, agile people could get me down, I'm sure of it, but I have no cell service, my phone fell into a mud puddle after my last fall on the same hillside, and how would I explain this?

Where would I begin?

Hi, I am on some rocky mountainside near the road. I've fallen three times, and this time, I cracked my head and jaw on a giant boulder when my hiking pole slipped. I fell because I have brain cancer, and my balance sucks. What was I doing? Well,

6

I'm on a quest to find the thirteen tunnels on the North Bend Rail Trail before I die.

But what if the EMTs had been exposed to Covid? There's no way I wanted to get it myself or give it to my parents. The good news is I am injured and stuck outside of the county, so no one I know would hear about it on the scanner, or the Ritchie County Gossip Radio. If this happened in Harrisville, my parents, my mom's friends, and everyone my dad had ever taught in school would know about it before I made it home.

I decide I need to get down this mountain on my own, but I'm going to have to roll and crawl; there is no way I can fall again. I'm hurt enough.

I scoot my ass through the mud and rocks until my backside bleeds through my pants. As someone who played roller derby for a long time and endured my share of rink rash, this bothers me way less than hitting my face on sharp rocks.

I talk to myself to see how much my jaw hurts.

I'm going to make it down this mountain I'm going to make it down this mountain I'm going to make it down this mountain.

Okay.

I can still speak.

Encouragement.

I never tell my parents where I am going; this is mostly out of resentment that I have to live with them, but perhaps this is also stupid of me. I don't think they will even miss me if I am gone a few extra hours.

I can finally reach the hiking pole; the other pole bounced at least twenty feet away, so I use it as a goalpost.

I will make it to that damn hiking pole then reevaluate.

Like a child who can't yet walk but feels bored with crawling, I scooch toward the hiking pole and use the other one to save my good hand, the left one. I'm a mess, but I'm still trying.

7

Maybe if I can get close to the road, I can flag someone down and get some actual help.

I parked at a church on the way up—when I asked the lady next door if I could park there, she yelled, *Erryone else do it, so you can too, hon! Don mind the dog, he just barks.* A tiny wiener dog yelped at me like I was yanking his miniature legs off, but he didn't move toward me or the road, thankfully.

Maybe the lady would be on the porch again and would help me. I don't live in West Union, but I could explain how I was, indeed, from West Virginia and *not* an outsider. If I told her my mom sometimes ventured over to this county to administer EBT cards, she might find me extra trustworthy and extend both hands instead of one.

Not that the lady needs an EBT card or has ever applied for one, but my mom's job adds an extra bit of ethos to my character; although I haven't lived in WV for a long time, people can trust me if I'm The Food Stamp Lady's Daughter.

But I don't see the lady or the dog.

I just keep scooching and bleeding.

Tunnel #6 was, by far, the easiest tunnel I've walked through, but the ingress and egress have been absolute bullshit. A deer frightened me on the way up the mountain, and I fell. I got lost on my way to the tunnel and added an extra mile to my hike, which caused a low blood sugar. (I thankfully brought granola bars and orange juice in my unstylish fanny pack my mother despises.)

And now I'm bloodily tumbling down a rocky mountainside (this is *not* an infamous WV rolling hill), without any security I'm actually going to make it back to my car.

I just keep making small goals. Toss the hiking pole. Roll a little bit. Stop and check out the sky above my bleeding head.

An hour-and-a-half later, I finally think I can stand again.

I can see my tiny purple Scion, which gives me hope.

However, standing is never easy. I try to maneuver myself toward the grass and away from the rocks, which have devastated me to this point. I am able to stand on the grass, but naturally, there's only a tiny patch and then more boulders. Though I have lost a great deal of trust in my good ol' hiking poles, I try them again. Paired with small, dancing sidesteps Jesco White would envy, I inch toward the base of the dirt mountain and nearly get run over because of course, I'm so excited to be alive, I am not paying attention to the cars.

This was my Everest, my K2.

I fucking did it.

I sit in my roller skate of a car and close my eyes. Is it the ankle-biter sausage doggo barking, or is The Mothman back for me? Did he follow me down the mountain, stalking me a bit before he decided to abduct me and my car?

He always chased people in their cars in the early days, you know.

I bet he was in that tunnel keeping me safe.

Me? I prefer the theory The Mothman was born a humble barred owl until he crawled into some unmarked nuclear liquids (which WV is also known for), took an unfortunate bath, and then rose above the hills like the Appalachian Jesus we didn't even know we needed.

Come save me, Mr. Mothman.

It's time to go.

PART I
#13

Boone, North Carolina

My mother, who believed she had a sinus infection, actually had a stroke.[1]

It is minor, as far as I can tell, but Jenifer Childers Samples has never been known for being entirely truthful or telling the full story.

After all, as a teenager I found the divorce papers in the attic from her brief starter marriage and straight up asked her about it. *Why is your first name on these papers, but your last name is P— and not Childers or Samples?* I knew it had to be her—she couldn't half-truth her way outta this one, not this time, because the papers clearly had *Jenifer-with-One-N* right there on them with a last name I didn't recognize, and everyone within a fifty-mile radius of my hometown knew my mom spelled the common first name in such a unique way.

Well, she said.

My sister Sarah, clearly too young to be hearing this but more excited than anyone to be lurking in the conversation, made a water droplet sound by flicking her finger to her cheek.

She had been perfecting this sound for weeks and at first, Jenifer-with-One-N looked to the ceiling as if we had an actual drip threatening the rickety white two-story my sister and I had carved our names into when no one was looking.

Well? I said and let a silence fill the room like the carbon monoxide that nearly killed us all a few years ago.

I was married once before. Your dad called him Pilgrim because he liked to wander.

She turned her head and walked away as dignified as Princess Diana, who was very popular at the time.

My dad *called him Pilgrim because he liked to wander?* Okay, good one, Ted. So, he cheated on her, obviously, but I wanted, needed more details.

When my parents were out, I took my own pilgrimage to the attic and surreptitiously dug through hundreds of old papers and clippings. I found the wedding photos. (That hat, Mom. Really?) I found the invitations. I found the remnants of My Mother's Life Before Children.

This might have bothered some kids, but this humanized her to me. She spent evenings flitting off to church and claiming *she wasn't as perfect as Jesus, but she wanted to be the next best thing.* I had no idea what Jenifer looked like without makeup; I'm not sure my sister or father did either.

But this! A husband before my sister and I existed? This proved she had been scandalous. She had made a few mistakes.

Jenifer-with-One-N Childers P— Samples was, actually, imperfect.

This delighted me.

But anyway.

The stroke.

I ring Dave, whom I reconnected with recently, after 20 years of knowing each other but losing touch. We are currently dating, or whatever we are calling it. Dave doesn't like to put

14

labels on relationships. He isn't working because The Pandemic has put everything on hold. He has time for me now, which, according to him, is perfect because he just hasn't had the proper time for me in the past.

This seems to be a recurring theme in my life.

Time.

I simultaneously have too much and never enough.

My mom had a stroke, I tell him, and my voice cracks. *I need you to get me home.*

One Month Earlier

Winston-Salem, North Carolina

The MRIs continue, but there is no remission.

My doctors don't say *no evidence of disease.*

I've noticed medical professionals are very cautious about using these words and phrases when referring to brain cancer.

Most of the time, they just slap the MRI results up on the screen and say, *This is your brain now.* Then they point to the other slide, the one with the giant octopus, cat hairball tumor. *This was your brain on drugs.*

Okay, that's not what they say but something close.

Everything since my surgery, chemo, and Jason Vorhees-mask radiation nightmare has looked normal. Well, normal except that now my frontal lobe has a black tunnel of its own with no light at either end.

Normal.

Everyone would like to believe I am in remission, though. Isn't that what happens when you finish surgery, chemo, and radiation?

Remission. No evidence of disease. Cancer free.

Well, sadly, that's not always what happens, especially when the cancer is all in your head.

Boone, North Carolina

CK is having trouble letting this abusive relationship go.

She has cried to everyone in Boone and beyond that I made everything up. She would *never* push someone into a wall, *especially a disabled person* and *especially when her best friend works for a domestic violence shelter!*

Three weeks before my mom's stroke, CK texts me she wants her stuff back, so I put everything on my porch.

Everything.

Her things, gifts she gave me, everything.

I want nothing to remind me of her.

I simply text her back a time she can pick the stuff up.

I am not physically able to get everything in one trip, but I try.

I accidently drop the teapot she gave me as a birthday or Christmas gift (it's not that I forgot; my birthday and Christmas are too close together and after *everything happened* three days after my birthday, I would rather just scratch December off the calendar altogether), and the ceramic mostly shatters on the concrete.

This feels great.

This feels fantastic.

This feels so wildly cathartic that I pick up the robin-egg blue edges and ram them into the pavement with all the gusto I have left in me, which is surprisingly, quite a fuckload. I keep smashing pieces of the love teapot until there's nothing left of our relationship but microscopic shards of glass I can't even feel with my good foot.

Suddenly, CK's vehicle rumbles down the driveway,

spraying gravel toward the abandoned apartment complex beside my building. I've thought about moving in there; I'm relatively sure no one would notice. Upon peeking in the windows, everything is still furnished and much nicer than the chairs and futon I own.

Last autumn *before everything happened*, I sat on the porch of number 13 and read *House of Leaves*. Trying to ground myself after a breakup with a narcissist and figure out if and how I still existed, I yearned to disappear in Danielewski's Five and a Half Minute Hallway, but the closest I came was having him follow me on Instagram after tagging a shot of the postmodern masterpiece in a Clarendon-filtered post.

For someone who wanted to disappear, I felt so seen.

That is until Danielewski instantly unfollowed my account after I followed him back but whatever.

I had my moment.

I turn to get back inside before CK sees me; it certainly wasn't my plan for her to witness me smashing the teapot. I was trying, for once in my life, to have a mature breakup.

To be nice.

To be fair.

To be civil, even if she did push me into a wall.

After all, I had told no one about The Incident, not at this point. I had kept my mouth shut because look, I did not want to ruin CK's life. She did what she did, but I was moving. We all knew that. I was never playing roller derby again. She was. I was leaving Boone, at some point, and she was staying put.

I was keeping my mouth shut.

It was for the best.

As I turn to go inside, I nearly lose my balance; my balance has been shit *since everything happened*, but I grab the doorframe and save myself.

Something drips from my head.

I did not fall, so it can't be blood.

I have this intrusive thought that although it's been nearly three years, my craniotomy scar opened like a cave and blood has started sweating out of the old, familiar wound.

This is it.

This is the end.

But first, I have to get inside before CK sees me.

I will sweep up the teapot bones at a later time.

When I get inside, I notice liquid all over me.

My hair.

My forehead.

My clothes.

The pug.

The fucking pug.

The people who live above me do not take care of their dog. Let me get one thing straight—I have no problem with pugs. I find their little squishy faces adorable. My colleague and friend Peaches has two pugs, Olive and Opal, and they might be two of my closest friends I've never met. This isn't the pug's fault, but the people who own the dog just let it wander out onto the porch above me and piss and shit whenever it would like.

A few of those times happen to be when I'm standing on my own basement-level porch.

There was also the time they threw the bong water out onto my own dog's fur, and she smelled like feet and cat piss for two weeks (no matter how many times I bathed her), but I forgave them of that.

But anyway.

I have bigger problems than pug pee and rank bong water.

CK, who typically moves extremely quickly, has decided to take her time getting her few belongings into her Kia. I really want to get into the goddamn shower and wash this pug pee off my skin, but I'm not making myself more vulnerable than necessary until I hear the Kia rumble out of Foscoe and down the road toward Boone.

I do not fucking trust her.

And I have good reason not to.

While she's there, I get a text from Dollfin, CK's ex who helped me tremendously when I first received my diagnosis.

I know where this is headed.

I witnessed CK treat Dollfin horribly when they dated; the first girl Dollfin fell for, CK led her on, and then once they were in an actual relationship, did things like scream at her for not being able to find her own work shirt and then found it exactly where she left it. *She always does this. It's fine,* Dollfin said to me with tears in her eyes.

CK says you've been contacting her, Dollfin's text reads. *You know how hard this breakup has been for her. You should leave her alone, you know?*

I want to scream I want to scream I want to scream.

I can still hear CK rustling around on my porch like the squirrels do at night when I'm staring into imaginary black holes and wondering if my next craniotomy will be worse than the last. Will there be more swelling or less? Will it be longer than eight hours? Who will hold my hand?

Nearly everyone is gone.

I take a quiet breath; surely CK has seen my tiny purple Scion and witnessed me awkwardly scuttle back into the apartment, but I don't want her to know I am here.

She texted me. She wanted her stuff back. I was trying to be nice.

I toss my phone onto the carpet, and it flies across the floor and taps the doorframe.

I suddenly don't care if CK hears me.

I realize with quiet intensity: I am getting stronger.

. . .

19

Boone, North Carolina

The phone calls begin very early in the morning.

I have always hated talking on the phone.

I answer because I am afraid something is wrong, something bad, very bad has happened.

Lately, I have taken to sleeping on the futon in my living room instead of the bed. Minimal light gets in through the front door, and I like it this way. I can sleep until noon or whenever, and no one notices.

Is this because of brain cancer or depression?

Probably both.

I've gained forty pounds since my diagnosis. I assumed I would just eat a bunch of delicious food and then die before I had to worry about the extra weight. Sadly, for my self-esteem, that's not what happened. Now I have minimal movement, a major sugar addiction, a face as big as a balloon, and strange early morning phone calls.

Hello?

Who is Don –?

I am not awake enough to understand what is happening; I recognize Dave's voice on the phone, but I have no idea who Don is. Do I even know a Don?

Don?

You know exactly what I'm fucking talking about, Suzanne. Don't act like you don't know.

I really have no idea.

I have no idea.

Don't play this cute little game with me.

Dave's anger intensifies like a boiling kettle. I'm fully awake now and ready to do damage control. Last week, Dave told me he didn't want to label our relationship because *we were two fully grown adults and didn't need to play that kind of game.*

I guess I misunderstood and thought he liked games; it's easy to see why this happened.

I should hang up the phone and never speak to him again; however, after CK alienated me from nearly everyone in my roller derby circle, I need someone to trust.

Someone all about me.

It's not a game. I don't know this Don person you're talking about.

Oh really, Suzanne? Well, you fucking should because he loved one of your cat pictures on Facebook last night around 1:15 a.m.

And then I do recognize the name. I didn't at first because he's a roller derby ref, and I've never known or referred to him by his government name.

He loved the picture because he has the same type of cat I do. We aren't close. We both like cats. He was married to one of my friends. There is absolutely no flirting or anything sexual going on there. He's just a nice guy.

Bullshit, Suzanne, Dave says. I can actually feel his spit coming through the phone. *Bullshit.*

I'm not lying. We are friends because he's a derby ref, and we both like cats. That's it.

You fucking cheating bitch!

Dave growls like a hungry wolf and ends the call.

I am so confused.

I haven't had coffee yet.

I know I've done nothing wrong, but I'm upset and feel horrible because Dave is clearly angry, and it seems to be my fault.

I've done nothing wrong I've done nothing wrong I've done nothing wrong.

He's going to eat me alive way before the brain cancer.

I call him back. I want to end this stupid argument.

I am better than this.

He is better than this.

We are better than this.

Dave and I have both been through too much to let some silly argument about social media get the best of our relationship.

Or whatever it is since he refuses to label it.

He answers, but he doesn't speak.

The silence echoes like all those years he stopped answering my letters and emails; I quit sending them when I learned he got married. How could I ruin that? I told myself it wasn't me after all. He was supposed to be with someone else.

Uhhh are you there? I ask awkwardly.

Oh, I'm here, Suzanne.

There's no love when he says my name; it's clipped syllables like bullets from a gun.

Look, we are adults here. I'm not going to let you talk to me like that. It's disrespectful, and I can't stop someone from liking a cat picture I post on Facebook. And why does it matter? It means nothing. It's a cat picture.

He hangs up on me.

I don't care.

I am proud of myself. Instead of blowing up like a grenade, I calmly approached the problem and reasonably stated my case.

I especially think that as someone missing a chunk of my brain and as a brain tumor patient on a seizure medication with a reputation for causing people to have a bad temper, I have done a bang-up job here. I didn't even raise my voice.

I fall back asleep.

I don't dream much anymore.

I would feel guilty.

. . .

Boone, North Carolina

The phone buzzes again, and I answer.

Dave. Of course.

If these phone calls were chatty and kind, I would welcome them. Instead, my phone has become a little ticking time bomb, exploding whenever his name pops up on my screen.

Hello?

I try to be normal. I don't want him to accuse me of sounding weird.

Listen, we need to talk about that little outburst you just had.

I am genuinely confused.

Outburst? Are you referring to the phone call we had earlier today? Because that certainly wasn't an outburst. That's called communication.

Communication my ass. You need to get your shit together and stop blaming your brain cancer problems on me. I'm not your brain cancer punching bag, Suzanne! I've said this before, but you didn't listen. This has got to stop!

Uhhh, I simply told you that you can't be mad at me for someone liking a cat picture—you know what? Never mind.

This will never be productive, not when he's in this kind of mood, whatever kind of mood this is.

Oh, never mind? You wanna tell Facebook boys like Don never mind? Well, I'm a man, and you're not going to tell men like me, men like me who shot Osama Bin Laden in the head for you, how I can talk to you. I can talk to you however I damn well please.

I am a compass of emotions right now and it's all going south, but of all things, I start to laugh. I can't help it. This verbal war with Dave has so many strange maneuvers; I imagine him with one of those yellow legal pads in front of him, the same kind he once wrote me loving letters on, making little boxes and designs to keep his story straight.

Facebook.

Brain Cancer Punching Bag.

Boys Named Don.

Shooting Osama Bin Laden in the Head, with a bunch of stars around it.

I AM A WHITE MAN AND CAN DO WHATEVER I WANT.

As long as you're being reasonable, yep, sure, I say. *You can talk to me however you want.*

I don't know why I'm continuing the conversation or the relationship, however he wants to define or undefine it.

Someone, most notably my parents, should have ended all this when I was sixteen and he started grooming me with cards and letters. I had no idea what grooming meant at the time; at 16, I was thrilled for someone to pay attention to me. I so often felt isolated and misunderstood in this little town because I focused on academics rather than boyfriends or football games. Dave was the only person in the outside world who contacted me, and he stayed regular in his communication. I could predict the afternoons when I arrived home from school when one of those yellow legal pad letters would be waiting for me in the mailbox.

Those letters were so exotic to a bored West Virginia teenager that they might as well have been tickets to Bali.

Now I see those letters, the same letters I ended up burning one day in college after he had his daughter and got married, as nothing more than manipulation.

In the mid-1990s, maybe some places had internet, but tiny towns like Harrisville, West Virginia, were shielded from instant messages, virus-filled chatrooms, and dolphin porn videos[2] until the late 90s and early 2000s. In the mid-90s, my sister and I were thrilled to finally have access to basic cable and VH1. Before that, it was only country music television. MTV was as far away as Myrtle Beach, which, as every West Virginian knows, is the vacation mecca of The Mountain State. I didn't know MTV existed until my cousin Kyle somehow located it on our grandmother's television.

But anyway, Dave is mad I have an opinion about how he treats me.

I don't have to be reasonable because I saved this country from terrorists, Suzanne. I can speak however I want. And if you want to put that on Facebook or in one of those little stupid books you write, you will be hearing from my attorney. His name is something something something and his number is something something something.

At this point, I lose it. His attorney's name sounds too much like James P. Albini, who was Michael Scott's trusted attorney on *The Office.* I cackle. I laugh. I don't care who hears me.

Are you...laughing at a goddamn war hero, Suzanne?

I halt my giggling troops for a moment.

I don't care if you're a war hero or villain. This shit you're trying to pull is absolutely hilarious. You're just trying to control me. This has nothing to do with you being in Iraq. You're just being abusive and trying to get away with it.

The call ends.

I go about my day.

I've got papers to grade.

Boone, North Carolina

I just feel like you need some sort of proof, Chris tells me. *Did the Petcube record CK pushing you into this wall?*

Is she serious right now?

She is.

I shouldn't be surprised; after dating Chris for as long as I did, she loved to say I *was making up stories* when I accused her of cheating on me. Of course, a month later, or a year later when she confessed to multiple salacious happenings I knew about all along, these stories were much more nonfiction than she let on. She was still pissed when I mentioned in *Frontal Matter* she cheated.

I didn't even want to bring up the whole being pushed into a wall thing, but since CK went all town crier and told everyone I lost my mind, CK had to get her lethal lesbian prattle into the mix.

The L Word was a fun show to watch for a reason.

I don't need anyone to believe me, I say. *I know what happened, and I'm leaving Boone. I just never want to see her again. Not now, not ever.*

She says you keep texting her.

I do not. She texted me to get her stuff, and I told her when she could get it. That's it.

It's very odd for people in abusive relationships to text their abuser—this just isn't—

Jesus Christ, it's actually not odd at all, and I don't block people like her because I want to know what she's going to do. And I never called her abusive, I just said she pushed me into a wall, which she did. Remember when she showed up completely wasted at my house at 3 a.m. when I was teaching the next day? And then she ended up kicking shit around my apartment, screaming at me for half the night, and when I finally got her in my car, she tried to jump out and kill herself on the highway? Then she threw her keys at the Fruits and Veggies Stand and called the police to pick her up but acted like someone else did it? She's out of control. I'm seriously freaking out here because everyone is acting like I did something wrong when I'm just trying to take care of myself, and that is hard enough right now.

But did the Petcube—

No! It records in present time. You have to pay monthly if you want it to keep recordings.

I don't think you're going to be able to prove this, quite honestly, Chris says. *It's very farfetched.*

I'm not even trying to prove anything. I just want it to be over. I just want to leave Boone. I just—I never want to see CK again. Look, I never really loved her. I never even liked her. I know that sounds horrible, and in a strange way, I'm grateful for the things she did for me. How could I not be? But...it just wasn't there, and I couldn't make it be there. I wanted to break up with her, and honestly, that should be okay. I tried to do it gently. I tried to do it nicely.

You know, Chris says, *honestly, you're right this time.*

Thank you.

I finally feel heard.

I was not the nicest person to Chris in our 306 (approximate) breakups, but I was nice, kind even, to CK. In my weakest physical moments, I still tried to help. I still tried to give her the benefit of the doubt. I still looked at her and said, *you are young. You still have time to learn,* even after she destroyed my cousin Kyle's house with a toilet paper party and bad mood.

But I don't know, Chris continues. *You're so unpredictable.*

I sigh. I should end the call now. It's not going to go in my direction. When I first started dating CK, she hated Chris. I understood. I had been a jealous girlfriend before, so I got it. I really did. I thought introducing them would fix things, would help CK feel more secure about everything.

I was doing my best here.

And then they became BFF, and I was the problem.

I AM UNPREDICTABLE BECAUSE I HAVE BRAIN CANCER AND AM MISSING PART OF MY FRONTAL

27

LOBE OKKKKKK AND I DON'T EVEN THINK I AM WRONG BY MOST PEOPLE'S STANDARDS ABOUT 98 % OF THE TIME.

I don't say that; I just think it.

No one says anything.

Uhhhh, Buckle?

This is a pet name. She knows better.

I don't think we can talk about this until you believe me, I finally say.

I deserve to be believed, even if I think I don't need it.

The bruise on my thigh from where I fell into the basket before I was pushed into the wall might be the only one to agree with me, but I'll take it.

Boone, North Carolina

Dave decides to visit, despite the threat of Covid. I know he will be cautious; he is the most meticulous person I have ever met. Still, the reunion feels frivolous, and I seem stupid for letting it happen.

Although she's still flitting around NYC, my sister tells me this in no uncertain terms.

Sarah and her ol' buddy Blaze Danger stop talking and start trolling. They sign me up for all of Donald Trump's mailing lists. They sign me up for Christian dating sites. They sign me up for KKK notifications.[3]

They sign me up for everything I hate.

She also sends Dave a message decrying he's *a child predator* because he wrote me letters when I was 16 and he was 25.

Sarah and CK must also be in contact because CK writes Dave a Facebook message noting she's the same age he was when he started penning me letters, and his daughter is the age

I was—how would he feel if she did the same thing to his daughter?

She's not wrong, and I think this is why he explodes.

Unfortunately, he takes all this out on me in his early morning phone calls before he arrives in Boone.

Do you know I'm an Iraqi war veteran, Suzanne? Do you know I was killing Osama bin Laden[4] for you? For you? And this is how you treat me? Your stupid fucking sister and your ex are sending me Facebook messages telling me I am a child predator when I was out there shooting high-powered Iraqis in the head, all for you, Suzanne!

I don't know if I keep my cool because I am different now or because I am just tired of drama altogether.

I...I have nothing to do with this. My sister and CK are doing this all on their own, and I can't stop them. I'm not speaking to either one of them right now. I stopped talking to CK after she pushed me, and I just texted her to get her stuff, and my sister—

This is all your fucking fault, Suzanne. Fix it. Fix it now.

I really have nothing to do with this. They are doing this on their own. You know I wouldn't call you a child predator; I wanted you—

Fix it, you fucking bitch. You know what? I'm tired of being your brain cancer punching bag. It's not my fucking fault you got cancer, but you act like it is. Dammit, Suzanne. This is all your fault, you bitch.

Thankfully, he hangs up.

I don't understand how this derailed into him being my *brain cancer punching bag*. Nothing in the conversation happened because of my cancer. It all occurred because of the carousel of people in my life who can't keep their shit together for a single second, and I'm honestly quite sick of it.

My arm shakes, and I am afraid I might have a seizure, but I don't. It's just nerves.

I try to make sense of the illogical. Brain cancer punching bag? I've never once yelled at him or even said anything untoward, especially about my cancer. CK is mad at me because I broke up with her, and my sister took her side. I don't control their brains or actions.

He calls back three minutes later, and I hold the phone a ruler's length away from my face. I have learned to do this to avoid damaging my hearing.

In three minutes, Dave has become a different person.

I'm sorry. You know I didn't mean any of that. It's just been hard lately with me being out of work because of Covid. You know I love you. I always have. I always will.

I should just hang up on him, but I soften. He has PTSD. He's been through a lot. He killed people in Iraq, and I don't understand any of that. How could I?

I get it, I say. *It's...it's fine.*

After all, this feels like my last chance.

A text comes in from CK.

I think about you all the time.

But anyway, Dave decides to visit, and he asks if he should bring anything. I don't know if this is a good idea, but I want it to happen. What if I die before Covid ends and I never find out if Dave was truly *the one* for me? What if? What fucking if?

Some board games and Starburst, I tell him.

Do you burn candles? he asks.

Yeah, why? Do you have allergies or something? I don't have to burn them.

I'm still accommodating.

I make them. I'll bring you some.

* * *

30

Dave shows up two weeks later with four board games, a giant bag of Starburst, and a candle called Meerkat Skat. So far, he is doing everything right.

Well, I'm not thinking about the early morning phone calls and naming a candle Meerkat Skat.

I've forgiven him for the anomalies.

Maybe the meerkat ate some berries.

Dave and I play a detective-themed board game where it's helpful to keep track of the other player's movements; however, he fails to tell me this when he gives me the instructions. He watches my game token and makes scrupulous notes on a yellow legal pad. I didn't know I needed to do this. He didn't really explain the rules, and it's clear I'm losing.

As I watch him note my movements, I remember the letters he sent me when I was 16. His ephemera arrived pre-internet, and I have always hated talking on the phone. He used the same yellow legal pads, always, and had the neatness of a serial killer, which if I remember correctly, was one of his interests.

He wanted to be an FBI profiler, and as a 16-year-old, I thought this was the coolest thing in the world, that a future FBI profiler was writing me, Suzanne Samples, someone who did baton twirling and read books in her spare time.

Now, I know exactly what he's doing.

Dave thinks he's smarter than I am. He wants to manipulate me. He, in his simple mind, believes because I have cancer and am nine years younger than him, can push and push and push me, and I'll just do whatever he says. He thinks because I believed in soulmates 20 some odd years ago, I still do.

I easily lose the game.

Dave smugly grins and makes circles around certain notes. I don't know what they mean, but I don't care.

I am on my best behavior.

I have been for a long time now.

I have a sinking feeling thing might not work out with my little soulmate here, but I'm still moving to Harrisville, and since most people in Boone either a) hate me because they believe I made up lies about CK being physically abusive to a disabled person or b) they have work commitments, I need to play this game a little longer so I can convince someone to move my shit and drive the U-Haul to Harrisville.

Jenifer Childers Samples didn't raise someone who can't manipulate others for the greater good of the community at large. At my best, I am quite Kantian.

You're really good at that game, I say. *It's just like I remember you; you were so into the FBI profiling stuff, and you could always read people so well. Including me.*

Are you hungry? Dave asks.

I know he believes me.

To him, I'm still the sweet 16-year-old who lives down the street.

Which is fucking disgusting, quite honestly.

Dave has been promising me *the best salmon ever.* I love salmon, so the bar is high. He swears he is a fantastic cook, and he will not let me down.

The accompanying asparagus is as small and limp as his dick.

This is my fault, of course.

I bought the asparagus and salmon through a grocery delivery service so I wouldn't have to go to the store.

Because cancer.

Because disability.

Because Covid.

But the limp asparagus and bland salmon is my fault because I acquired it a day too early. I should have thought it through better, he tells me. I should have just let him go to the store and pick it up because he is the knight in shining fucking armor, and no one can do anything as perfectly as him.

I eat the entire meal so I don't piss him off, and besides, I've given insulin for everything anyway. I even throw in a couple Starburst at the end because he brought those, and I know it will make him happy.

He wants us to read a play aloud, just the two of us.

I refuse.

I've had enough for the night.

C'mon, he goads me. *It will be therapeutic.*

I don't like plays.

I'm not lying—drama is my least favorite genre of literature. Sure, I enjoy seeing the occasional stage production, but reading them for class? Fuck that shit. I could not do it and tried to avoid classes that focused on plays at all costs. The last thing I wanted to do was a dramatic reenactment of some play he brought with him.

You'll like this one, he says.

Did you write it?

The only reason I ask is because if he did, I know my cousin Emily and I will ridicule the writing later. Is this mean? Absolutely. Does he deserve it? On all accounts.

Nope, Dave says as he pulls out two copies of a play called *Gruesome Playground Injuries* by Rajiv Joseph. He won't tell me the summary of the play and demands we jump into a table read.

I don't want to do it.

You don't have to voice the characters like I do, just read the play in your normal voice. It's fine.

I admit, I am intrigued by the title.

The work follows two friends, Kayleen and Doug, as they pass through one another's lives over the span of 30 years. The title is literal and metaphorical; there are the

33

disgusting injuries described in sparse, grisly detail, and there's the deeper cuts, and that's why, once I finally agree to read the work aloud, I cry through the entire experience.

I knew you'd be into it, Dave says, morphing back into his regular voice again.

It did take me by surprise, I say as I wipe my face with a stray paper towel.

And I am back in Dave's clutches once again.

I know exactly why he chose this particular play. Sure, it's been more like 20-some years with us, but with each scene, I could picture myself as Kayleen and Dave as Doug. Sure, Kayleen and Doug are the same age and Dave is nine years older than I am, but I could visualize the unrealized love between Doug and Kayleen and see it resting on the table between myself and Dave.

Here we are, after all this time.

How could I let a few weird phone calls get in the way?

Boone, North Carolina

I brush my teeth and feel like I might fall.

I hear gravel spitting into the lawn.

I peek and see a vehicle the color of CK's rolling down the driveway.

I check my phone.

My sister.

Do you really think it's a good idea to have Dave visit you during a fucking pandemic when you have cancer, Suzanne?

I don't know what you're talking about.

Since Dave and I have reconnected and Sarah sent him the Child Predator Message, my sister has been pushing me away faster than my friends did when they found out I had cancer. I feel like she's jealous I finally found my soulmate, and she hasn't.

It's so obvious.

CK is over there right now and told me she saw his car.

WHY IS SHE STALKING ME?

Another text comes through. Dave has wandered off to the bathroom.

It's Dollfin.

You really need to stop texting CK.

I'm not texting her. Not at all.

She says you are.

I cannot fucking win.

Dave is going to give you Covid, and you're going to die.

My sister won't shut up.

Dave comes out of the bathroom and hugs me. He has arms as sturdy as ancient tree trunks, and I feel protected. I finally start to relax. For a moment, everything is quiet. He leads me to the bedroom, and I am excited scared freaking the fuck out oh my god if my sixteen-year-old self could experience this! What would I think if I could see the future! This is living this is life this is what I have been waiting for pure ecstasy the best a soulmate what I have always wanted.

Dave kisses like a lizard.

I let it go.

Okay, I don't.

This is the worst kiss of my life.

I might throw up, and I haven't puked in a very long time.

No one says anything.

This. Is. So. Awkward.

I'm able to have sex, I say. The awkwardness has to be about my disability. I know it. Dave feels afraid to fuck me because he sees me as fragile.

Okay then. I guess you should take off your clothes.

He goes into the bathroom. I don't know what he's doing in there. Maybe looking at porn because I'm not attractive? I get it, and I'm totally okay with it. I've gained a lot of weight since my diagnosis. Cancer doesn't make everyone skinny.

He doesn't come out of the bathroom for a long time.

I'm afraid to know.

I shed my clothes like the lizard who kissed me might molt. I try to shed my clothes, anyway. I'm still slow, heavy, and lethargic, but I'm finally naked. Suddenly very insecure, I toss a blanket over my body. Dave has yet to emerge from the bathroom.

I grab my phone and play some Candy Crush.

I'm on level 4,345.

When he opens the bathroom door, Dave is naked and has a problem with my kitten Delilah.

This damn cat is ruining everything. She's so annoying. Why would you want a cat like that?

I'm suddenly way more protective of my kitten than turned on by Dave.

She's not even three months old yet. Of course, she's going to be wild. She was rescued with 30 other cats from underneath a house.

Her name isn't Delilah; it's Banshee. I'm renaming her.

Well, she's my cat, so you can't rename her.

Dave inches closer to me on the bed and gives me another hug; he seems to have forgotten about Delilah, but I want to find her and hold her close to me so no one can hurt her.

Are we going to do this or what? he asks.

Yeah, yeah, of course, I say as he gets on top of me.

I already know I don't want to do this, but it's easier to realize this upon reflection. At the time, I honestly thought Dave was my *last hope for love,* and I needed to, had to make everything work. Unfortunately, because of the whole paralysis debacle, my legs won't spread like the good girl he wants me to be, and Dave doesn't like this.

He gets frustrated.

Stand up, he commands.

I don't know if I can.

Stand up. We will make this work.

Hold the bed. I can't get inside you if you're on your back. Your vagina is fucked up. It's not like other women's. It doesn't work the way it should.

I want to cry, but I don't want to give anyone's small dick the satisfaction of my tears.

When he is finally inside of my *fucked-up vagina,* he grabs my cheek and yells, *Who's fucking you? Who's fucking you, Suzanne? Who is it? It's Dave. Dave's fucking you. Say it. Dave is fucking you.*

I don't say a word.

I see a Kia driving up the gravel.

I am terrified of everyone right now.

Boone, North Carolina

Dave needs to go outside to make a phone call.

I struggle to dress myself, but I am tired and dirty and strange. There was no cuddling afterward, no affection.

I've had more affection from stray cats.

I wonder who the phone call is from, but it's not my business.

But then my mind drifts to double standards. How would Dave react if I took a phone call directly after we had sex? He would lose his mind, scream, and maybe even throw shit.

I am on level 4,348 of Candy Crush.

Dave has disappeared for over 20 minutes. The phone call

could be from his daughter, which would be fine. Absolutely acceptable. I would encourage that phone call.

However, I've never heard him discuss friends, aside from his ex-wife. He tells me they *have a great relationship*, and I'm never to question their dynamic. After all, they *have a child together,* a child who is almost an adult, and because I don't have a child with anyone, I simply *could never understand.*

So, I don't question anything.

Thirty minutes later, he comes back inside after his phone call and tells me it's *a friend from theater group.* No more details than that.

Instead of the mysterious phone call, Dave wants to talk about his ex-wife.

I listen to story after story about how he met his ex-wife, the time they spent together, how they raised their daughter, and all the fun they had. I'm truly unbothered. Everyone has a past, and everyone has a right to discuss that past.[5]

I speak up.

Yeah, I think it's great you're still friends with her. It's nice to be friends with an ex. I still talk to a few—

Do you honestly think that's a good idea?

To be friends with exes? I mean, you just said—

It's different. We have a child together.

So? Your child is in high school now. I'm not saying you shouldn't talk, but honestly, you can stay friends with your exes, even if you don't have kids together.

I—Dave— can handle that, he says. His blue eyes turn the color of gravel. *I doubt you—*

Suzanne—can. And I have to worry about boys and girls with you.

But I love and care about you—

Oh, save it, Suzanne.

Look, it's you. It's always been you. If something happens with you, I'm not dating anyone else.

Bullshit.

I am on level 4,440 of Candy Crush.

I'm serious.

That's bullshit. How many men are you seeing right now?

Uhh...just you. I've told you that and given you no reason to disbelieve me.

Oh, you've given me plenty of reason.

Excuse me? I mean, let's be real. I have no issue with your ex-wife and am very glad you are friends and get along, but you just spent a really long time talking about her, and I'm giving you reasons to believe that I'm seeing someone else? Are you kidding me?

Pull out your phone. Now.

I am freaked out. I don't have a single suspicious message on my phone, but I don't know what he expects. I'm starting to understand how he can turn a *hi how are you* into a *I want to fuck you right now.*

Open Facebook.

I comply, and I fucking hate myself. I should have told him to leave right then, but I believed we were soulmates. I had loved him since I was sixteen. I had waited for this my entire life. My brain cancer nightmare was going to end in a beautiful dream of love, kindness, and acceptance.

I am so confused.

Okay, let's start from the beginning, Dave says. *Open your friends' list.*

I don't really know where this is headed. I am worried, but I'm not even sure what I'm worried about.

I sit on the bed as Dave peers over my shoulder and instructs me whom I can keep and whom I need to delete as my Facebook friend. Any woman? They can stay.[6]

He demands I delete guy after guy from my friends' list.

His eyes shoot bullets into my iPhone, and I honestly wish it would just morph into shrapnel so I could blow it from my hands and onto the brown carpet that needed replaced seven years ago.

I don't typically block or delete people from my social media; it's just not my style. Even if we haven't spoken for years, I'm not going to bounce them from my page. Why? It doesn't affect me if they stay.

But apparently, for whatever reason, it bothers Dave.

I stand up for certain male friends. People I work with? They stay. Travis? He isn't going anywhere, even if you want him to.

If Dave sees their profile and doesn't deem them a threat, he allows it.

Eventually, the sun sets, and we are only on the letter D.

I don't have fucking time for this, and I can't believe he does.

I can't believe anyone does.

I don't realize this at first, but he demanded every single man who wasn't white be booted.

Why did it take me so long to understand?

Why did it take so much?

I was in no way prepared for this.

The road from Boone to Harrisville

Dave packs the moving truck quickly, and I'm gone from Boone forever.

Things with Dave have been great the past three days. So amazing I've forgiven him for calling me every morning at 6 a.m. and accusing me of cheating on him because a friend on

Facebook, a friend I haven't seen in three years, "loved" one of my cat photos, or, Fogwoman[7] forbid, a photo I'm actually in.

He can't help it when he goes off like that. He has PTSD from killing the most important Iraqi leaders. He isn't like the other soldiers over there, he told me once on the phone. He did THE BIG THINGS. The things no one else wanted to do. He shot people, the scariest, worst enemies of America, in the head.

He did it for me.

He did it for you.

He did it for all of us.

Therefore, I have to forgive him. What else can I do? He's been through enough. He doesn't need me to make his life worse by sassing him or backtalking him during those 6 a.m. phone calls. He spent all that time in Iraq *putting his life on the line*, and how could I disrespect that? I would be absolutely remiss if I did.

And, as Dave reminds me, since I voted for Obama, I've already done enough horrible things throughout my adulthood. If I was still that sweet, conservative 16-year-old who lived down the street from him when he was 25, then we would have zero problems.

He has what he calls *retroactive relationship jealousy*. He explains to me that because of this, he will never get over my past relationships with other men. Whenever he tries to fuck me, lizard kiss me, or even hug me, he just imagines me with other men and cannot handle his rage. When he goes off, it's my fault.

I shouldn't have dated other men, ever.

I should have waited for him from when I was 16 to 38 and not let another male touch me.

Obviously.

I am the reason for his issues.

That's why I need to, therefore, delete all men from my Facebook.

Dave knows nothing about Instagram, and I cling to my Clarendon filter like it's a vintage-colored lifejacket.

I cannot speak to other men on social media, in front of him, or basically ever because of his retroactive relationship jealousy.

I am smart enough and still with it enough to understand there are major missing pieces here, but I am too afraid to move my game token forward. He's always watching, always noting my movements on that yellow legal pad.

I haven't spoken to my sister in weeks.

When I ask Dave during an apologetic phone call why he never contacted me after his divorce, he answers with silence.

I am at a loss.

If his relationship rage is all my fault, I have no idea how to fix it.

As he drives me from Boone to Harrisville in the smallest U-Haul available, Dave regales me with stories about his former work as a prison guard. As a true crime fan (but *not* the type where you drink a glass of wine and chat with your friend for two hours before you talk about a ten-minute case once you're already good and sloshed—more *Dateline: Uncovered* or *Generation Why* hardboiled true crime), I am interested in Dave's experience.

Oh, it was amazing. I mean, you had your boring stuff, you know, but every now and again, you'd get something good. Dave still has a slight Southern accent, which I find charming.

Genuinely interested, I ask about his most interesting prisoner.

Definitely the Virginia Tech cheerleader. I mean, she was smoking hot. Little blonde girl. Everybody wanted to search her, if you get what I'm saying, but I got to do it. Whew! Damn, that cheerleader body was something else. She was tan, too. She took care of herself, if you get what I mean. Not like you.

I stare at the bumpy road ahead of us. Now that I'm outside of my Boone apartment, I am putting together this puzzle of what a shitbird Dave is. Did he really just say that to me? I'm not jealous. I long ago, like when I was ten, gave up the dream of being a blonde, skinny cheerleader, but *she took care of herself, if you get what I mean. Not like you* bit was too far.

Way too far.

I have a problem with this statement in general. A woman can *take care of herself* and still be fat or far from a size two, and there's nothing wrong with either one. Taking care of yourself doesn't automatically mean you'll be skinny or tan or blonde or a cheerleader. It might, but it doesn't have to.

I also have a personal problem with this because Dave knows *taking care of myself* for the past few years has meant getting out of bed. Feeding myself. Giving myself insulin. Taking a shower.

Making sure I don't die.

Dave is Machiavellian enough to know exactly what he is doing; he wants to make me feel bad because he's mad about Facebook, which I ultimately find ridiculous and can't believe I gave into in the first place.

I consider the age gap. Dave is nine years older than I am and perhaps doesn't understand that for someone of the Oregon Trail Generation, Facebook is just a way to connect with people I actually don't talk to in real life. They can like or love all the pictures or statuses they want, and it is of very little consequence to anyone.

Except Dave, apparently.

Gatsby, who has been sleeping by my feet, barks and whimpers.

I don't bite.

I simply play along.

What did this sweet cheerleader do to get herself put in prison?

Who knows? Probably drugs.

Sounds like a pretty unique case. I'm surprised you don't remember.

I remember her waist. I would have liked to have held that waist up if I was a male cheerleader. Damn! And her curling iron. She brought her curling iron to jail. Can you believe that! At least she cares about the way she looks. Do you ever curl your hair?

I never fucking curl my hair. It's extremely straight, and that's fine by me. I like makeup, though. It's fun.

You know, I haven't seen you wear makeup a single time since you've been around me.

Well, I was more focused on spending time with you than putting on damn makeup.

When did you start talking like that? What happened to that sweet little Suzanne who lived down the street from me and always did her hair and makeup for high school?

I stare straight ahead on the road. We have at least four more hours. I'm going to vomit. This is too much.

That girl died a long time ago.

Harrisville, West Virginia

I cannot accurately tell you what is going on with my mother.

I don't think my father could tell you either.

Maybe her church could?

I know I have stepped into a very dysfunctional environment, and there is no whipping this U-Haul back to Boone.

· · ·

Harrisville, West Virginia

When we arrive at my parents' house, everyone is thrilled to see Dave, the hometown hero. Although he hasn't been to Harrisville in years, people here never forget anyone or anything.

Never.

Ever.

And if they do, there's always Jackie, the owner of The Pizza House, who will tell you anything you want to know and hand you a homemade cookie to satiate your hunger while she fills you in.

Dave's sister comes over to see him and help get my stuff into the house. We all mask up because at this point, no one knows much about Covid, and we especially don't want his sister to take anything home to her kids.

Dave doesn't seem especially close with his family anymore.

When Dave and I reconnected, I asked how often they saw each other. After all, he and his sister only live a state away from one another, and Dave's daughter is a teenager; he doesn't need to change her diaper or make sure she takes naps.

He gives me a vague answer of sorts, something to the effect of *it's been a few years, you know she's always busy. My sister is the busiest woman I know.*

I've always really liked his sister. She looks exactly like Elaine from *Seinfeld*, and there's not a sinister sinew in that woman's body.

While everyone talks outside, six feet apart, I slowly and carefully walk Gatsby around my parents' yard. For a 13-year-old dog, Gatsby pulls extremely hard, which it dangerous for me to walk her, but she has to go to the bathroom, and everyone else is too busy to help.

If I fall, I guess I fall.

The Midnight Cowboy, one of Harrisville's finest, has been mowing the yard for my parents, so at least everyone will be able to see me and hopefully help.

I don't fall, but I'm extremely tired. Cancer, long car rides, and 6 a.m. phone calls where I'm excoriated because random people love my Facebook cat pictures have exhausted me.

I just want to get inside and eat Pizza House pepperoni rolls.[8]

We were supposed to be moving into our new home, replete with a section for myself, Gatsby, and my two cats, but Covid happened, and understandably, everything got behind. Because of this, myself, Gatsby, and the cats, one of which was a former feral, will be sequestered in my tiny childhood bedroom until further notice.

I am sure that will go well.

It's still better than being in Boone, where most people believe I'm lying about CK's behavior and actions.

It's still better than hearing her car bounce up and down my isolated driveway.

It's still better than being peed on by a pug.

We finally decide to go into the living room and talk. Dave and his sister bring the futon inside; it's really the only heavy furniture item I own, and it's a gray, cheap, bendable number.

As everyone catches up, Gatsby has made herself center-stage on the blue carpet of my parents' doublewide. She's never been the type of dog to scoot her ass across the carpet, but there she goes, just like a little train engine, chugging along while everyone chats. To my horror, I realize she has chunks of shit stuck everywhere on her furry behind.

Welcome home!

Oh my god, Gatsby! I try to chase her and pick her up, but I'm not quite mobile enough. She's a smart dog and knows she's having a problem, but she cannot fix this herself: Gatsby needs help.

We all need help.

She darts around the living room, slinging brown poo all over the blue carpet.

Everyone either screams at me or does absolutely nothing but stare.

Suzanne, get her! Get your dog! Do something!

Okay, sure. There are people in this situation I do not expect to do anything. My dad and I have similar mobility problems, so I'm not imagining he's going to chase the pup and capture her. Dave's sister is just a visitor and came at the last minute to help, and she did this to be nice. I do not expect her to dirty her nice clothes she wore to school that day.

But my mom and Dave?

Why the fuck are they just standing there?

Why aren't they helping me?

I am not strong enough to catch Gatsby, nor am I able to pick her up. She may be 13, but oh Fogwoman, she is strong! She is spry! She has gone wolf wild in Harrisville!

I do my best to corner Gatsby so the shit is confined to a certain space of the doublewide. Sure, we are moving, but we don't know when the new home will be finished.

We might be smelling dog shit for a minute.

I finally trap Gatsby by the piano.

Not the piano! my mom screams.

I'm really tired of everyone yelling at me lately.

I get where my mom's coming from; it's a nice piano, and she loves it. Her mother was an excellent piano player, and they shared their love of music with one another.

But listen, Gatsby is *near* the piano, not *on* the piano.

Gatsby has not sat her shitty behind on the piano bench and pounded out a jazz number.

47

My mom's outburst scares Gatsby, who, of course, believes this is some type of really fun game. Gatsby darts to the gray futon, a symbol of her home in Boone, where everything was safe and not full of poop.

I grab her collar.

Waiting for Gatsby on the futon is none other than Princess Peppermint, a giant 23-pound matted marshmallow specimen of a cat who burns with the fire of Satan inside her and expresses this toward everyone but my father, who is only excused because he feeds her.

Princess Peppermint takes one look at her new nemesis, hisses a Latin curse at Gatsby, and empties her bowels on my gray futon.

Such a feline move.

Motherfucker.

My cats, still in their crates, stare at PP in complete horror and disgust. They would never pull such a stunt.

Well, Pru definitely would have, but she's been gone for a few months now.

My dad, suddenly energetic, finds paper towels from somewhere and gives them to me. I am now using Poop Dog Gatsby (the name is affectionate, don't worry) for stability, but when my dad tosses me the paper towels, I have to give up a hand.

Wait a minute.

I expected to clean up after Poop Dog, but everyone is staring at the futon.

I try to throw the paper towels to my mom.

I just got my nails done, she says as she fans out her hot pink fingernails with a rhinestone flower pattern on the fourth finger.

Those look great! Dave says.

I can't take it anymore.

You've got to be kidding me.

48

My dad reaches for the paper towels back and dabs the futon.

That's not how you do it, my mom says. *The paper towels should be wet.*

I'm doing my best, my dad grumbles.

My dad and I, the two disabled people in the room, are doing our best while everyone else stands there and admires my mom's new nails amidst the smell of animal feces.

Half standing, I pull Poop Dog to the bathroom; yet this is a very unsteady position for me, and I trip in the hallway. I suppose no one hears me, or no one cares.

I don't understand why Dave isn't helping me.

Isn't he supposed to be my partner? The one getting me through this? The one saving me from it all?

Instead of assisting me, he just stands there and stares.

Gatsby whines, and I pull myself up in the special way I formulated.

Knee knee hand hand left foot right foot downward dog inch together up.

Thanks for nothing, assholes.

I get Gatsby into the tub by lifting her left paws first and then hoisting her dirty butt into the shower.

I leave Gatsby, shut the door, and return to the living room with an old wet towel to clean up the poop. The others keep chatting about old neighbors, and it's like I'm already a ghost in my own family and with the guy who is supposed to be in love with me.

After I clean everything, I toss the dirty towel into a plastic bag, tie it up, and lob it into the yard into a graveyard of cardboard boxes.

I return to the bathroom and climb into the shower with Gatsby.

It's going to be a long night.

. . .

Harrisville, West Virginia

Dave thoroughly impresses my parents with his Army tales and professional job experience. His *yes ma'ams* and *no sirs* do not go unnoticed by Ted and Jenifer Samples. He entertains with his charismatic stories about helping our mutual neighbor with her lightbulbs because he was *the epitome of the boy next door* and well, everyone knew it, especially the neighbor who needed her lightbulbs changed by someone handsome and tall enough to complete the job.

Half the time she still had months, probably years, left on those bulbs, but I went over there and changed them anyway, Dave says.

His Southern accent is only barely noticeable, mostly when he says *I* and *light*.

My dad asks him about the putting hole his father tried to install when they lived in the red house next to us.

Oh, my gawd, he worked on that thing forever, and of course, I had to help him! Everyone else was gone, and I was the only kid left. I don't think he ever got it finished, but he hit golf balls into that thing anyway.

This is especially funny because there is a golf course half a mile away from us.

So, what was your time in the military like? My dad asks.

I am surprised; my dad might typically say a few sentences the entire day, and it's usually a hot take about music. Last time I was home it was *That Adele is a good singer, but she's not much to look at* and *Is that Carrie Underwood?* (It was Taylor Swift.) *I don't care who it is. It's not good. I'm tired of all these blonde country stars. I'm going to turn it off.*

Then he read a world atlas the rest of the afternoon.

Dave answers him with gusto. *Oh, it was great. I drove*

around officers and, you know, kept them happy. I got to hear a lot of their stories and opinions. I'll tell you, not a single Democrat in the bunch!

My mom and dad love this.

He knew they would.

I do not.

I am so confused.

Okay, look. I know very little about the military. The most I know is my dad's brother once pretended to be an Army General at a parade and was discovered by my dad's other brother, who ratted him out. The most I know is that it's extremely difficult. The most I know is I'm thankful for their service.

However, it doesn't take a General to figure out the person driving around officers isn't the same person shooting Osama Bin Laden in the head.

Also, I am in the minority with my political views at this table.

Still. Everyone is happy. Everyone is getting along. No one is yelling or mad about Facebook. My mom seems to be having a good day. My dad isn't complaining about the appearance of today's musical acts.

I have a break from trying to hold it all together with my defective brain.

I can tell my parents already see Dave as family. This feels right, I convince myself. We belong together. We always have.

I repeat this three times in my head until I almost believe it.

Ellenboro, West Virginia

After Dave helps me move my life into my parents' living room, we stay together at the Sleep Inn in Ellenboro, which is the next town over. Oil and gas have been discovered within the last few years, causing this community to erupt with more money and potential than this area has ever seen. People who were too poor to buy new clothes at the local Dollar Store suddenly found themselves sitting on millions of dollars in a *Beverly Hillbillies*-becomes-a-reality plot twist.

Naturally, as true Appalachians, most of the nouveau riche stayed in the area and gave away their money to charities or the people who weren't sitting on the same reserves of oil and gas.

That's just how people are around here, and I would be lying if I said I didn't miss them sometimes.

In the early 90s, the consolidated middle and high school were built in Ellenboro, and my class was the first to blaze through the 6th through 12th grade program. We didn't have the option of writing on the bathroom walls and not getting caught or Hacky Sacking inside for fear of someone's shoes scuffing the floor, but we had new shit, like sweet digital clocks and lunch tables without a giant rainbow of chewing gum decorating the underside.

There was a Dairy Queen a few tenths of a mile from the school, and that was it.

Now there's the Sleep Inn, a gambling joint disguised as a coffee shop (one of my dad's friends found this out the hard way), and the shining crown of the county, a McDonald's-Go Mart combo to fuel everyone's hamburger and gasoline needs before they abscond to Route 50.

My mom pays for Dave's room at The Sleep Inn, and I join him. I can't believe Jenifer allows this to happen. Despite being in my late 30s, she considers it a sin to sleep in the same bed with a man I'm not married to. If anyone saw me, and they certainly would, they could tell someone at her church or her friends.

She either really likes Dave, or she has given up.

Maybe a combination of both.

We arrive to The Sleep Inn around 7:30 p.m., and my old classmate checks us in. My mom told me my classmate once had a brain tumor herself, and I am sympathetically horrified. Is it something in the water here? There was the documentary about DuPont; the film showed how a farmer's animals near Parkersburg, the "city" thirty minutes down the road where we had to go see movies, go to Wal-Mart, and go to the WV fancy restaurants like Olive Garden, kept dying because the chemical plant dumped their water into the creek where his animals drank. A few years ago, Mark Ruffalo starred in the film *Dark Waters* that explored this theme further.

But I could accuse so many different entities for causing my cancer, and it's not going to matter.

Although I can barely walk from yesterday's turmoil, I go back out to Dave's car we towed on the back of the U-Haul and get my bag.

I didn't get enough for supper,[9] *so I'm going to McDonald's next door*, he announces.

I'm a little hurt. We just left my parents' house, and they were extremely accommodating to him. My mom paid him for moving me, bought the hotel room, and asked him about five different times if he needed anything else to eat.

Identical pickup trucks litter the parking lot like cigarette butts; once cleanly white, some of them are now brown and dirty with West Virginia mud.

What the hell is with all those trucks? Dave asks.

They are oil and gas workers.

Oh, yeah, I knew that. I wasn't asking you. Just thinking out loud. You good to get inside?

I'm an afterthought.

I'm good.

I guess it's going to be that type of night.

This is somehow my fault; I must have said or done some-

53

thing to fuck this up. I need to make this better. Dave is not happy, and this is somehow related to the time spent at my parents' house. Despite the love and admiration, they showed him and although my mom gave him way too much money for helping me out, something in his brain has turned these interactions negative. I dig into what's left of my brain and search for something I must have said.

Nothing.

The hotel room is Covid-pristine, complete with a condom for the remote control. I don't feel safe taking a shower on my own, so I scrub myself with some wipes. Of course, I'm hoping our interactions will be normal, and Dave will want to have sex or at least cuddle. Since my diagnosis, I have noticed people's fear of touching me. Not everyone, of course, but people who had no issue running up and hugging me *before everything happened* now like to keep an even ten feet away—and this was prior to Covid restrictions requiring six. I don't know if it's because people consider me fragile (although I certainly don't look fragile),[10] or if they are afraid, they might somehow catch brain cancer or become infected with the chemo or radiation I received.

Good news—it's all either flushed out in numerous hotel room toilets or trapped in my brain, where it's dying off and creating something called *radiation necrosis*.

This is the last time I will see Dave until we don't even know—he has not mentioned any future visits, and he refuses to tell me where he lives. I wanted to send him a card once, just like the old days, but he acted like he didn't hear me ask what his address was.

All I know is Roanoke.

I turn on the television through the remote-control rubber and find an episode of *Guy's Grocery Games*. I'm happy to know the remote-control stays protected from my cancerous body. It's a veteran-themed episode, so I feel confident this will turn Dave's sour mood around.

The door opens sooner than I expect, and Dave stands there with nothing but the key card.

You didn't get any food? I ask, though I know I should have stayed silent.

Well, Suzanne, the McDonald's closed early tonight, so Dave doesn't get dinner.

I—I'm sorry. I try to stay logical. *Did you try Dairy Queen?*

No, no, it's fine. Dave will just go hungry tonight. I've done it before. No need to worry about Dave.

I really just want to drive myself back to my parents' house, and that's saying a lot.

Dave uses the third person quite frequently when he's mad, and I'm not sure if this is some sort of narcissistic, selfish trait or he's experiencing a break from reality.

Maybe all the above.

Be patient be patient be patient.

He's been through a lot. No matter what he did in the Middle East, he's experienced some shit, and I need to respect that. Honor that. Revere that. I don't know what that must have been like or what he deals with now because of it.

Are you not going to take a shower before you get in bed? He walks into the room and notices my dry hair. *Dave doesn't like going to bed hungry or sleeping in dirty sheets.*

I swallow my spit. If Covid wasn't happening, I would take the elevator down to the lobby and hang out with my old classmate once I was sure Dave fell asleep. Facing my parents after the happy dinner would be too awkward. How could I explain this? Dave didn't feel like you gave him enough food, and he tried to go to the McGasoline[11] to get more. They were closed, and he didn't want anything from Dairy Queen. He came up to the room, started talking about himself in the third person, and then demanded I take a shower in the non-handicapped accessible tub.

I can't really get in that type of shower by myself, so I just wiped—

Well, it's a good thing Dave is here to help you. Take off your clothes, and I'll lift you in. Dave is strong.

I am humiliated I am scared I am locking up.

Most of my focal seizures occur when I am afraid.

About to fall? Arm starts shaking.

Nervous about election results? There goes my right foot.

Not super keen about Dave lifting me and putting me in the shower? The entire right side of my body quivers like it did when I was on the radiation table.

Once we are in the shower, everything changes. Dave sprays and washes my scarred body—from both surgery and falling— lovingly and gently and acts as if he has been given the most important task in the world. He adjusts the water to my liking and makes sure everything is in place so I do not fall. Exiting a non-accessible shower is always the most difficult task, but Dave puts his muscular biceps under my squeaky-clean armpits and pulls me from the bath like I'm an important weapon about to detonate.

He wouldn't dare drop me onto that floor.

I insist on dressing myself, even if it takes forty minutes. The extra weight has worsened my mobility, but I'm stuck thinking that I can't exercise at all. I did do some YouTube "Chair Yoga with Nancy" in Boone, but I don't know if I could count that as exercise.

Movement, maybe. Exercise, no.

Anyway.

Dave, despite not getting enough to eat tonight, seems to be in a better mood. I don't understand these switches, but I contribute everything to PTSD. Although I try, I wouldn't understand.

I have to be patient patient patient.

I'm an important weapon about to detonate.

Even if he yells at me, it's not him. When he calls me at 6 a.m. screaming, that's post-war Dave. When he talks about himself in the third person, that's someone I don't know and should just ignore.

We sleep beside one another in the hotel bed, but we don't touch. Neither of us tries. Guy Fieri's frosted tips cook me to sleep with roast beef recipes and the hope that the rest of my life, however much is left, won't be like this.

The remote control is the only one getting any action tonight.

This is the last time I will see Dave in person.

I'm an important weapon about to detonate.

Ellenboro, West Virginia

I've been driving my mom to physical therapy, and she seems to be doing well. She's having some problems with her vision, but her arms and legs are strong.

I usually don't admit wanting to be like my mother, but I'll take this trait.

Strong.

My dad always wants a cheeseburger from the McGasoline, which happens to be next door from the physical therapy center.

I did not get this trait: the ability to eat whatever and not gain weight. Later in the day, he'll have chocolate pudding, Mr. Bees potato chips,[12] pizza for dinner, and chocolate ice cream for a snack. One of his health issues is that he is perpetually underweight. He only exercises when my mom forces him to, and even then, he refuses to take his hands out of his pockets.

If you have time to stop at McDonald's, he always says.

He knows I'll have time.

A text from Dave lights up my phone while I'm in the drive-through: *What are you doing? I called and you didn't answer.*

I took my mom to PT, and I'm getting my dad a cheeseburger at McDonald's.

You're being shady, Suzanne.

The only people I still talk to in the area are my friend Jodi and cousin Amanda; I don't chat with any men from Ritchie County, and he knows this.

I'm not being fucking shady.

I'm helping my parents.

I'm being kind.

I'm being a good daughter.

If he wants to call that shady, then there is something deeply wrong with him I can't fix. I stop responding, and he doesn't like this. He calls over and over and over, until I find a pocket of the town where I don't get service. I can't take the sound of the vibrating phone anymore, but I know if I block him, he will find me. He will message me on Facebook or email me. He will Facebook message my mom, who adores him and has no idea about his temper. I haven't mentioned anything to her; she is trying to recover, and I feel bad enough she had to pay to bring me home to help her.

I have to forgive him. I don't have a choice, and he knows this. I will never, as he has told me, find anyone who loves me like he does. He has known me forever, even if we didn't speak for years. He is the only one who will *accept me like this*, my brain filled with disgusting foreign growths, making me untouchable to anyone but him (and apparently, sometimes him). I have to stay with him *because he understands.* He is the only one who will tolerate my issues and problems, the only one who will put up with being my *brain cancer punching bag.*

I need to accept Dave's issues, his problems. After all, as he has mentioned, I have contributed to these issues and problems by voting the wrong people into office, dating the wrong people when he wasn't around, and handling his PTSD the wrong way.

Oh, and by picking up my father a cheeseburger at the McGasoline drive-through.

HOW DARE I.

Wrong wrong wrong.

I go back to the physical therapy center to pick up my mom, but she's not ready.

Dave calls again, and though I don't want to, I pick up.

You have to stop this, I say with a steady tone. *You can't treat me like I'm doing something wrong when I'm just helping my parents out. That's ridiculous. I am in the car alone, waiting for my mom.*

I haven't always been this chill. After everything I've been through, I just don't have the energy right now to throw temper tantrums like I once did. I could blame it on being short, being a Sagittarius, being full of feminist rage, or all the above, but does it matter? I just don't care enough to fight anymore.

I don't fucking know that, now do I, Suzanne? How am I supposed to know that no one is in the car with you right now? You're probably fucking someone right now, and I'd never know.

This is so preposterous I have to laugh. Not a single person wants to fuck me, not even Dave. When he had the chance, he ridiculed my vagina and body-shamed me. Why would he think anyone else would want me?

I have to go, I say, and it has nothing to do with Dave. The physical therapist walks my mom out to the car. She looks as

59

pale as my dad's McGasoline cheeseburger bun and can barely stand on her own.

Does she need to go to the emergency room? I ask, very concerned.

She just needs more Gatorade and maybe some sugar! the therapist says.

I don't know what to do. What if she passes out? I can't lift her up, and neither can my dad. My mother is extremely thin, but my dad and I are weak as fuck. If she was in the emergency room, my mom would be safe.

Don't we all just want to be safe?

Are you having a low blood sugar? I ask my mom as the therapist helps her into the car.

I am the worst person in emergency situations. Honestly, it's probably a good thing I am the one with brain cancer and diabetes because I wouldn't know what to do if one of my loved ones had this happen to them.

However, if my mom is having a low blood sugar, I can fix this.

It's difficult seeing her not have power over her life. For the last 37 years, I've seen her control, well, everything.

She seems to perk up once we are back in the car. I offer to return to the McGasoline and get her a milkshake, something she tolerates well despite her Crohn's disease. She agrees, and we head there. I wonder if Dave has somehow installed a GPS tracking device on my car; I'd hate for him to accuse me of *being shady* again.

To be fair, in some ways, the McGasoline is kind of a shady place. Truckers know it's the only place between Clarksburg and Parkersburg to get any type of food and fuel. Route 50 is a lonely road; Sarah and I even saw an apparition on the median there late one night.

A man with a hat a man with a hat a man with a hat.

Suzanne? Did you see that? My sister asked me years ago.

I gripped the steering wheel of my '92 teal Pontiac Sunbird. *Fuck.*

The horn started beeping on its own, and we both screamed.

It's fine, it's fine. You know the horn does that.

The apparition disappeared.

We know what we saw.

My mom agrees to a milkshake, and I know this is a good thing. This will, for sure, get her blood sugar up. If it's something else, then I don't know what to do.

Hi, can I get a large vanilla shake?

The ice cream machine is—

You all know the rest.

We go across the street to Dairy Queen, which my mom says *is no McDonald's but will do.*

By the time we make it home, I have 13 missed calls.

Harrisville, West Virginia

Dave is going to buy me a house.

He tells me to look on Zillow or wherever else I want. Since he's not working, he will find the properties, check them out, take some pictures, and let me know what he thinks. When I say I can't do this because I don't have any money saved for a down payment—cancer not only wiped out my left frontal lobe but also my checking, savings, and the $20 worth of bitcoin I impulsively purchased because *what if*—he tells me not to worry. He can take care of this because he can get a VA loan, which will be zero dollars down. As long as he is working and can afford the mortgage, I can work to satisfy myself. If I want to cut down on my class load, fine with him. Teach one class a semester? No issue. Not work at all? Great!

I honestly didn't know this option existed, and now I feel extremely lucky; someone wants to buy me a house. I quickly begin searching Roanoke for available houses and find an affordable one story with a hot tub on the back porch.

I send him the link.

I've been on that road. The driveway is too steep.

Okay.

I find a brick ranch-style house with a basement; Dave mentioned he needed a basement to make his candles.[13]

That one looks like it's very close to neighbors.

Okay.

I'll just look and let you know what I find.

Okay.

I redirect my search efforts and look up roller derby teams in Roanoke. I will never play again, but I am sure that some team in the general area would love to have an extra volunteer. I express this to Dave.

Why would you want to do that? You have me.

I decide I will just do it without telling him. He acts in one of the community theater troupes in Roanoke, so I can leverage my roller derby hobby with that. You want to do community theater? I get to do roller derby.

I don't realize how I am oversimplifying this. Clearly, Dave will do whatever he wants while I sit at home like the good little undefined whatever he wants me to be.

He asks me over and over when I am going to move to Roanoke, and this irritates me. For one, my parents need me right now, and he knows this. I can't just pick up and move when I am the only one able to drive. My mom's stroke caused vision cuts, and my dad, in addition to the aftereffects of Lyme disease and Parkinson's, has severe cataracts requiring surgery. I can't move to Roanoke right now. Two, although builders should have finished the new house weeks ago, it isn't done and my two cats, Gatsby, the litter box, and I are cooped up in my childhood bedroom until they finish.

My parents blame Princess Peppermint, but I wonder if my mom just wants another way to control me.

This seems to be a theme with people in my life lately.

Also, I don't know how Dave expects me to make another move during Covid. This trek to West Virginia was necessary; a move to Roanoke would not be.

But I'm the one who loves you, Dave says on the phone. *Sure, your parents love you in a way, but not the same that I do. I was meant to take care of you. Right now, you're taking care of them, but you have cancer.*

I know, I say, considering his words. Dave is right, kind of. I am taking care of them, and I do have cancer just waiting to return. This is probably too much for me. I shouldn't be doing this. But then again, what else could I do? I can't go back to Boone. There's an entire roller derby team who thinks I'm lying about an abusive relationship. I can't depend on one or two friends to constantly bring me groceries, so I don't have to leave the apartment and risk constant Covid exposure. Harrisville, with more farm animals than people, is the safest place for me right now, even if I do fall asleep to the scent of cat shit each night.

As my mom says on every phone call, *Suzanne is here! We wanted her to move home so we could take care of her, but she's taking care of us now.* She says this in front of me as if I can't hear her, or maybe she just doesn't care.

I feel trapped I feel trapped I feel trapped.

So do my cats.

Living with Dave and sneaking off to roller derby events while he gallivants off to theater practice seems very appealing because of my current situation. Would he even realize? Would

I try to hide this? Probably not. I am not good at hiding anything.

Of course, there is the new house problem. My parents created a wing in the place just for me. Sure, it's small, but it's a matter of principle. Sure, I asked my mom *if I were to leave, would that be okay?* and she said, *Yes. If you start feeling okay and want to leave, fine by me,* but was that passive-aggressive? Jenifer is known for her passive-aggressiveness, but this seemed rather genuine. I wouldn't want to move to Roanoke before the completion of the home; that would be absurd.

I need a date, Suzanne, Dave insists.

I can't give you one right now. You know why. There's a global pandemic, for crying out loud. It wouldn't be safe for anyone if we tried to buy a house in Roanoke right now.

I'm doing this for us.

I appreciate that, for sure. But we have to be patient. We've waited this long, and I don't even know why.

You know what? he says. *I'm going to go.*

I...didn't mean to make you angry.

I've angered plenty of people since my diagnosis; this is nothing new. However, it's rare for the mad person to avoid telling me why they are angry. Typically, they are more than happy to let loose on me and explain why I've pissed them off.

Dave is different, in so many ways.

I'm just not sure all those ways are good.

Winston-Salem, the Dash, North Carolina

I'm back, bitches.

Although I'm one of many scared shitless by Covid, I'm still required to drive to Winston-Salem for my MRIs and oncology appointments. The hospitals have yet to shut down, and as long as no one has a temperature, cough, alienesque complexion, or strange fainting spell,[14] appointments run normally.

Winston-Salem is two hours from Roanoke.

It's been about two months since I've seen Dave.

Instead of the five hours from Roanoke to Harrisville, I am hopeful perhaps we could split the two-hour difference; on my way back home, I could drive an extra hour to meet him. Or, I could just drive two more hours to Roanoke and stay with him. Or, OR! He could just meet me at my hotel in Winston-Salem.

This seems like the perfect opportunity to get together. He still isn't working because of Covid, and I'm obviously still teaching online. As long as my MRI is good, I would love nothing more than to see his home, hang out with him, and get to know the present-era Dave a bit better. Despite the horrible phone calls, I still have hope as he says, *we have always been soulmates.*

I'm not ready to give up, not on my life or this relationship.

Once I get to my hotel parking lot, I try a soft request through a text. I've learned to avoid the phone calls.

Hey! I'm driving to my MRI in Winston-Salem and didn't realize that it was so close to Roanoke. We should meet up!

Naturally, I'm hoping Dave will lessen the burden on me and offer to drive to my hotel. He's told me that although he isn't working, he's getting unemployment and *wasn't hurting for money anyway.* Okay, then. It should not be a big deal to dump some gas in the tank and do a quick visit. I know that because of the pandemic this might seem entitled, but according to Dave, all he has done is drive around and check out future houses for us. He has not exposed himself to anyone or anything. Also, this is my Last Chance for Love, and pandemic or not, I want to give this relationship the best of what I have left, even if I am missing a giant chunk of my frontal lobe.

I enter the hotel lobby and am ready to relax before the big day and DoorDash some North Carolina cuisine.

FUCKING BOJANGLES.

To make MRIs more tolerable and since I've been able to save money by moving in with my parents, I decide to splurge on 3-star hotels instead of Motel 6s. I'm not expecting great things, but I'm expecting good.

Sadly, my room smells like an old school bus with a cigarette-addicted driver.

I toss my bag on the floor. I don't want to risk going back to the front desk and re-exposing myself to potential Covid germs. I, for sure, don't want to be a Karen. I also just paid too much money for a hotel room that smells like a bad elementary school memory.

I hold the hotel room phone six inches from my ear.

Front desk.

Hey, this is Suzanne in Room 312. I...I hate to be like this, but my room smells funky.

I'll send up Steve.

I have no idea who Steve is, but he shows up a minute later without a mask and makes himself at home on the chair. With his tucked-in collared shirt, chinos, and spit-shined shoes, Steve looks more like a high school basketball coach than a hotel manager, but if he's going to get me a different room, I'm all for it.

Coach Steve sniffs the air.

Good god. What happened in here?

I miss North Carolina.

Couldn't tell you.

I'm going to put you in 314.

I let him stand and get six feet ahead of me before I follow him to 314.

The new room smells more like a clean bus, so I deal.

I check my phone.

Nothing from Dave.

I'm starting to get irritated. I've expressed to him how difficult MRIs are; even if things seem fine, even if things seem as if they are on the upswing, there's always a chance the oncologist can look at you solemnly an hour after the MRI and say, *things didn't look good,* or *there is a suspicious spot on the film,* or something of the sort. The last time I spoke to Dave about the upcoming MRI, he was shocked to learn brain MRIs come back with results so quickly.

That's not how they work, he mansplains to me. *I've had plenty of MRIs for my knee, and it takes at least a week for the doctor to get the results.*

It's a brain MRI, and I have brain cancer, I say. *It's a little different.*

Are you trying to say my knee isn't important?

That's not what I'm saying at all—it's just—

I can't win.

I hop in the hotel bed and order my Bojangles; it's probably going to be the only thing to look forward to this trip, but it's enough. I watch a TV documentary about Travis the Chimp, and though I'm familiar with the story, I'm not any less horrified when Travis rips off a woman's face for holding his Tickle Me Elmo toy.

I start crying, quietly at first and then sobbing so loudly I'm afraid Coach Steve might come up and check on me. Travis didn't mean to hurt anyone, and that woman didn't deserve what he did to her. People should not keep exotic animals as pets, especially ones known for ripping off faces and hands.

Travis wanted to protect what he loved, and he died because of it.

How many times have we all wanted to protect what we loved?

How many times have we almost died doing it?

How can we blame Travis?

In my weak moment, I decide to text Dave again. I always try to avoid double texting people; it never works out. It's been over an hour, but maybe he's working out or in the shower or seeing his daughter. He usually tells me what he's up to, and I thought he would be slightly more concerned about me today, but he's not. While he's usually blowing up my phone and making certain I'm not texting or letting other men 'like' my Facebook posts (because, somehow, I should have control over that), today of all days, he's as silent as a funeral.

Look, you know MRI trips are really hard for me. I'm alone in this hotel and would really like to see you. I was hoping we could meet up.

I realize with the sadness of a chimp missing my favorite toy, I am frightfully alone.

Sure, I would not expect anyone to visit me in this hotel because of Covid, but there's not even anyone I can text. My sister is mad at me because of my relationship with Dave. My roller derby family thinks I've slandered CK for abuse and has cut me off. I haven't spoken to most of my true friends, what few are left, for fear Dave has somehow tapped my phone and will stop talking to me because he will believe I am in love with any and all of them.

I have to worry about both guys and girls with you.

At the time, I took it as a flirtatious statement; he found me attractive and knew I was bi, so he believed everyone else would find me attractive as well.

Looking back, I realize how naïve this was.

He just wanted to control me.

Of course, Dave has not tapped my phone, but I found myself in such a precarious state, I thought anything might be true.

The woman Travis the Chimp attempted to slaughter is still alive today. After multiple facial replacement surgeries, she still speaks about the horror she faced that afternoon. She and her family took Travis' mother to court but eventually reached a settlement when the former friend died.

Suddenly, my brain cancer issues and loss of friendships don't seem so terrible.

My fucking Bojangles arrives early, and I eat more than any common person would believe a cancer patient could.

Still nothing from Dave, and I actually start to panic. For someone who constantly checks in on me, this isn't like him to disappear. Was he in a car wreck while looking at houses for our future plans? He had mentioned potential high blood pressure in a couple of calls. (No kidding. I'm sure the constant screaming has nothing to do with it.) Did he have a heart attack? Was his daughter okay? Was she in a car wreck? Did she have some sort of health issue?

His daughter wants to be a writer and works in a coffee shop. Although I've never met her, I feel an affinity, not like she's a daughter or even a stepdaughter, but more like she could be a favorite student of mine. I once sent her a recording of how to submit short stories for publication. I didn't show my face or anything because I didn't want it to be weird, but Dave said I should do it; it would be helpful.

I want to be helpful.

I take a Klonopin to fall asleep early.

I need to be up and at the MRI building by 7:45 a.m.

Dave still hasn't texted or called.

Instead of worrying about MRI results, I fret over Dave and Google "red flags in a relationship" and "signs of a controlling partner."

If you have to Google it, you already know.

I fall asleep in the middle of checking each number on the list.

They isolate you from loved ones.

I think of my sister, who was once my biggest fan but can't stand Dave.

Check.

They criticize or body shame you.

I think of my apparently weird vagina.

Check.

You feel the need to report to them, and when you don't, you know you will be punished.

Shit.

I don't need to list the others.

You already know.

Wake Forest Baptist Health, the Dash, Winston-Salem, North Carolina

I am relieved to see Caleb, my favorite nurse, waiting for me after I check in. He's the only one who gets my IVs on the first try. Whenever I tell the others *I'm a hard stick*, they roll their eyes and say something to the effect of *everyone thinks that*, and then they try to get that shit in my arm and become as baffled as an English teacher trying to draw blood with a pencil.

I just smirk as they bruise me up.

I don't mind.

The bruises remind me of roller derby.

I'm so sorry, they all say. *Let me go get Insert Name of Other Tech Who is Better at IVs.*

But Caleb is an IV inserting wizard. He's a prodigy with the needle. He's an expert with his tools.

It's easy, he says. *You just need confidence.*

And I am confident in him, which is why this relationship works.

I have a few of these casual friendships now—people in the underground city of the hospital who recognize me. It's sweet how they never forget. I always assume they will, but it's nice to know how much medical professionals truly care. Once, one of my former nurses approached me in the lunch area to tell me she was happy to see me and glad I was up and walking.

I nearly cried.

After Caleb expertly inserts my IV, the woman who always tells me I *smell clean, which is awesome because most people in a hospital don't smell like that* helps me onto the table.

They never play music for the MRIs here, but there is a picture of a puppy, a kitten, and a flower.

It's something.

Then I wait.

The Wake Forest Baptist Cancer Center, a place I've come to know as the Wal-Mart of cancer care, a one-stop shop for anyone and everyone's cancer needs, bustles as usual. Everyone is at least wearing masks, which most in my hometown have failed to do.

I see Dr. Stroupe and hour later.

Your MRI looks boring! he tells me. *Which is great news.*

I beam. How do I keep doing this? How is this even possible? I don't even care.

I am alive.

I am breathing.

I am ready for more fucking Bojangles tonight.

I finally look at my phone when I sit in my tiny Scion.

Nothing.

No text from Dave, no call.

I've come to understand he only calls when he wants to yell at me.

71

Now I am angry.

Although my MRI went well—very well in fact—I needed Dave's support, and he abandoned me. I feel just as I did when I was 16, and he was writing me letters but dating someone else he would eventually knock up. If I had done this to him, even if it was just over a missed call on a regular day, he would have called and called and called and called again until I had no choice but to answer.

I was trying to be polite and normal.

I was trying to be understanding.

I was trying not to be a goddamn psychopath.

This, though, is unacceptable.

Each MRI could mean the glioblastoma has returned, that I'm actually done for good.

I've had enough.

I flex my texting anger.

Where the hell are you? I've had a really hard time doing this MRI by myself. How would you feel if you had brain cancer, and I didn't text you back? How would you feel if I showed up in a town close to you and didn't answer your texts?

I'm so frustrated I pound the steering wheel and scream.

I've done this in my car too many times now.

The phone rings in the middle of my scream.

I weakly answer.

Hello?

He has me right where he wants me.

After my boring MRI, I should feel thrilled right now. Ecstatic. Celebratory. Jubilant.

Instead, I feel like I want to sink into the rubber protection of my tiny Scion tires, which are, in fact, the biggest part of the car.

Dramatic, I know.

Do you want to know why I haven't been answering you, Suzanne? Do you really even have to ask?

I am too exhausted for this.

The six-hour drive, Coach Steve, crying in the shower, the MRI, Travis the Chimp, crying in the shower again, another six-hour drive in my future.

I needed you, I say. *I needed you, and you weren't there. You're all I have.*

I know that, Suzanne. And guess what? If you keep this up, you're not going to have me, and you'll really be alone.

Keep what up?

You know what.

I really have no idea what the fuck he's talking about. I have not noticed anyone suspicious liking or loving any of my Facebook posts. Surely, he doesn't know about my Instagram. I stayed alone and lonely the entire time I was in The Dash, except for Coach Steve. Were they somehow friends and he knew Coach Steve sat in the room in my chair? I'm so paranoid about the smallest things.

No.

There is absolutely nothing that could have made him angry.

Did my sister send you another message calling you a child predator? I ask and almost make myself laugh.

I still love my sister.

I don't care if she hates me.

Well, Dave begins, *the night before you left for your little MRI, I was browsing your Facebook profile pictures, and there it was. A picture of you, a little white girl, and that goddamn — from 2009. You want to know why I never contacted you? THAT'S why I never contacted you. You were fucking a goddamn –.*

He used that word.

73

That word.

I can tell Dave has used the word so many times, it's just part of his vernacular. He gives zero fucks.

He gives zero fucks about it, but I've had enough.

This is not okay.

First of all, you need to stop using that fucking word. It is not okay. Never say it again. Ever. It's unacceptable in any context.

Oh, and you think it's okay for a little white girl like you to date one?

Yeah, I sure fucking do. You know what? I don't regret dating him at all. He's a really nice person. We broke up because we weren't right for each other and wanted different things. Not because he's Black and I'm white. He's a great guy and has an adorable family now. I'm still friends with him, and that's okay. I want the best for him. If you don't like that, that's your problem. Also, that's an old picture from over a decade ago I didn't delete because I had no reason to; it was part of my life that was bothering no one until you came along. You went through A DECADE of Facebook pictures until you found something that pissed you off, and then you chose to throw it at me during a really stressful time.

Dave ended the call somewhere in the middle of the necessary tirade.

A day later, the drive back to West Virginia goes faster because I'm still so fucking pissed off.

Harrisville, West Virginia

My parents don't ask about the MRI.

They never mention my cancer, surgery, or anything related to any of it.

Well, that's not entirely true.

Your hair came back really dark, my dad says.

He is color blind.

It's always been that dark, I tell him. He just hasn't seen me for years because even if my mom visited North Carolina, which she only did for very special occasions, like other people's weddings, my dad didn't come. He hates to travel. They came to visit me once, right before my favorite cat Pru passed away, but I was bald.

But anyway, since the MRI was thankfully boring, I don't have any news to share.

Sometimes I am so disinterested I sit (very carefully) on my parents' front stoop and watch the deer cross the main road. The creatures have infiltrated town and become domestic outdoor pets. Not many care if they destroy gardens. Two snowy white deer,[15] Powder and Puff, remain the favorites. My dad and I joke we should sit at a card table outside and charge five dollars per person for those who come to gawk at our beloved outdoor friends.

Our neighbor Mary Beth calls to me when she hops out of her vehicle.

Hey, how was your MRI?

She had seen me before I left and asked me where I was headed.

I am glad to know someone cares.

It was boring, which is good! I yell.

Great to hear!

That's all it takes.

Harrisville, WV

I have heard nothing from Dave since he yelled at me for having an undeleted Facebook picture from 2009. I am no longer sad about this.

I am still fucking pissed off.

Just when I think he's going to leave me alone, Dave texts.

I'm texting you in the morning, just like you always asked me to.

He's not wrong. I have asked him to do this, but I expected his texts to be gentle and sweet. The *good morning* text everyone wants. Not a belligerent, resentful *I'm doing this because you asked* text.

Good morning!

I decide to try.

I don't know why, except that I am awfully desperate.

I slept in The Americana Room last night. It's actually the spare bedroom, but I'm tired of smelling cat shit first thing in the morning. My mom decorated The Americana Room with flags and teddy bears decked out in patriotic outfits. My grandfather's Burial Flag sets proudly on a shelf above the bed. There are red, white, and blue Longaberger baskets my mom earned from selling them before the company went bankrupt. Somehow, Jenifer beat the multi-level marketing system and actually made money from doing this.

I can see Dave's old little red house from The Americana Room, and it takes me back. It's now a psychiatrist's office, and I sometimes wonder if I could get an appointment just so I could see his old bedroom and feel the love and excitement of my teenage years again.

I don't know why you wanted me to text you.

I lose the will to try very quickly.

Text wall time.

Because I want to have an adult relationship with no drama, but you're showing me you aren't cut out for that. If you're not mad about something that happens on social media, it seems you want nothing to do with me. You stonewalled me during my MRI and were doing absolutely nothing that seemed important. I wanted to meet up with you then because we weren't that far from each other. I needed you, but you were nowhere to be found and had no good excuse. You have a rage problem that you can't control. I don't understand what you've been through, but you constantly blame me for my "outbursts," when in reality, you're the one having them, and over things that don't actually matter. This makes zero sense.

Oh, I have a rage problem?

You sure do.

Although I still fall all the time, I am finally starting to grow my mental legs back. I don't know why I'm putting up with people who physically or verbally abuse me. I've had enough, and I'm going to fight harder than ever now. Just like glioblastomas can grow tentacles, my courage grows enough to scare a Cthulhu.

My only problem right now is you.

And then, looking at the little red house that is now a shrink's office, I text the meanest thing I've ever said to anyone.

I wish you were the one with brain cancer.

I immediately regret it. Although I basically wish Dave the worst, I don't wish anyone *that* worst. However, I must show you, the reader, I sink low sometimes, and this is a new low. I've never thought this about anyone. Hell, I've never even wished diabetes on anyone.

Instead of blue, the text I sent Dave is green.

To confirm my suspicion, I try to call and am sent straight to voicemail.

He has blocked me.

I'll never know if he actually got the text, but to this day, I hope he didn't.

I didn't mean it.

I am on level 4,678 of Candy Crush.

I am not crying at all.

I am surprised at my lack of emotion. Dave has worn me

down to nothing. I feel nothing nothing nothing. I have nothing left to feel; I am done.

My phone rings.

I don't answer.

It rings again.

Without looking at the screen, I answer.

I know it's him.

WHAT.

We have been trying to reach you about extending your car warranty!

I hysterically laugh.

I don't think I'm okay.

I'm on level 4,680 of Candy Crush.

The phone rings again again again.

I don't answer.

One more time, like a bad 80s song.

I say nothing.

You know why – date little white girls like you? Because you give them status and mean nothing. They want to tear you apart with their giant dicks. They want to—

That's not how it was. You don't know because you weren't there. That's not what it was like at all.

You need to quit having these little outbursts, Dave screams. *You know what? We are going to give this other personality of yours a name, or you and I are never going to work.*

He is absolutely right about this. We aren't going to work because I am done. If I would ever get the chance to speak, I would tell him this.

Dave continues.

I had a counselor once who told me that naming things like this could be helpful. You like paranormal stuff. What about Zozo, the name of the evil entity that comes out of the Ouija board and won't leave people alone? I bet Zozo would keep

78

fucking a –, Suzanne. Don't you think? You should thank me for being with someone like you, with your fucked-up pussy and brain cancer, Suzanne!

I scream.

I fucking lose it.

I can't take anymore.

I let loose directly into the phone, a wail Zozo would be proud of.

I only answer to myself, the Fogwoman, and Zozo now.

This time, I end the call.

My dad, who lost a lot of his hearing as he got older, is already on his way back to my bedroom because he could hear Dave screaming obscenities at me through the phone; he was that loud. My parents, who think War Hero Dave is the only Dave who exists, know nothing of his yelling and constant verbal abuse.

Suzanne? My dad asks, clearly in a panic.

I don't know what to say or do.

I'm still in my pajamas and am not usually awake yet.

I... I'm not okay, I say.

Dave is no longer on the phone and has finally stopped his constant calls.

I'll get your mom, he says. *She's with Michelle.*

Oh god. This reminds me of the time when I got really sick while visiting my parents during Christmas break from college. I started vomiting and couldn't stop. I knew the puking happened because I started my period, but I didn't want to talk about it. My dad, the only one at home, wouldn't stop asking me why I was so sick.

I sat by the toilet and projected yellow bile from my gut and answered as he asked a million questions through the door.

Suzanne, did you eat something?

No, vomit.

Is your blood sugar high?

No, puke.

Do you have a virus or something?

Noooooo thepukeandvomitblendtogether.

Well, what's going on?

I started my period.

I'll get your mom.

And here we are again.

No, no, it's okay, I'm just...it's fine. I don't want to put more stress on my mom. She's been doing well, and our family friend Michelle took her for a walk.

I know what to do.

I text my sister.

I was so wrong, I type. *I was stupid. Dave is the worst. You were right.*

It's only 8 a.m., but I predict Sarah will be up from the night before. If she tests negative for Covid, she's coming home for a week before she moves to Texas from NYC. I'd been dreading her visit; our relationship had suffered interminably since I started *doing whatever* with Dave, and I knew Sarah and I would be avoiding one another in our childhood home, which, with all my shit in the living room, did not have the space for us to be dodging each other like bumper cars. She and our mom both have big personalities, while my dad and I are a bit quieter and have no issue blending into the pale, luminescent wallpaper and couch[16] that resembles the "Jazz Cups," popular in the 90s, with the turquoise and purple squiggle marks.

Still, it's a small space.

I'll be home in an hour, she texts. *It's been crazy. Had to rent three cars, lost some of my clothes, thought I might be murdered by a redneck on a backroad in rural NY. Thought I might have the Covid antibodies but I DON'T!!!!!! Still gonna take a shower as soon as I walk in the door. I've got three burner phones with me. We will take care of Dave.*

We're back, bitches.

Wait.

Why does Sarah have three burner phones?

I don't have time to think about it. My mom arrives home from hanging out with Michelle and is ready to hear the tea. Jenifer Childers Samples may not know how to deal with cancer or MRIs, but she's not going to let a guy, even an Iraqi War Hero, trample all over her oldest daughter's heart.

This is a crisis she can deal with.

What is going on?

To see my mom, no one would ever know she had a stroke. She still looks like she's in her 40's, and she knows it. As one of the crew administering EBT cards for the people of Ritchie County, West Virginia, she takes no shit.

My mom is the only person I've ever feared.

I can't lie to her; I never can.

I'm done with Dave. It's over.

What happened?

I am surprised I am not crying, but I feel lighter. Free. Like I just had a different type of tumor removed.

Well, I say, *honestly, he's just not a good person.*

I don't even know where to start.

Is he messed up from the war?

Uhhh... That's part of it, but I don't think that's all of it. I think he's just got a lot of weird ideas about women that don't align with me and who I am as a person. And he's really racist.

That's the most concise way I can say it.

Okay, she says. *Do you want to go for a walk?*

Yep, but first I need to burn a few things.

Most people think living in West Virginia means you are missing teeth and walking around barefoot all the time. First off, that's not always true, but who cares if it is? Secondly, living in West Virginia really means you always have access to burn piles in the summer.

If you don't have your own burn pile or share a community burn pile with your neighbors or friends, you aren't living your best West Virginia life.

I collect two items.

An Army t-shirt Dave flung at me the one time he visited in Boone; gray with a mock neck and super long, I found the shirt horribly uncomfortable and an outdated, high-schoolish practice: *We are dating (or whatever), so wear my shirt so people know you belong to me!*

A Beatles poster, still shrink-wrapped in plastic with cardboard behind it, that he gave me during a Christmas when I was still in high school. This was after he moved back to Virginia, and we'd been writing letters for over a year but before he married. I'll never forget how he proudly marched into his parents' living room of the little red house with the gift, my face beaming because he remembered me and what I liked.

I didn't care about any of that now; I wanted to watch it all go up in flames between our house and his old home.

Harrisville, West Virginia

As expected, Sarah shows up around 2 a.m., jacked on cigs, Mountain Dew, and maybe cocaine. Her circus dogs caper about the doublewide without a single care and pee in all the corners.

She calls to me from the laundry room in a small, weak voice.

Suuzzzzzzannnne. I need a big towel.

We all forget she agreed to dump her dirty clothes in the laundry room in case she somehow had Covid fleas on her. It seems silly to say now, but this was when we were all wiping down our grocery bags in case the virus could be carried on scraps of paper.

No one knew any better.

Despite being in her 30s but still partying like a teenager, Sarah is somehow the most modest person I know. Although both my parents are asleep, she would never walk through the house to our shared bathroom in her bra and undies. *Someone might see her.* The neighbors have been asleep for about six hours, but they might be waking up soon.

I nearly trip over the tiny circus dogs as I rush to the bathroom to get her a fluffy towel to hide all 98 pounds of her body.

Claire licks my leg. Jared lifts his own leg and pisses a bit on my foot.

It's good to see them.

Harrisville, West Virginia

It's noon, and I am anxious for Sarah to wake up.

I am not permitted to bother her; if I do, Claire will rip my fingers off.

We have work to do today.

Dave has already started harassing me on Facebook. I've done my share of harassing exes on Facebook, so I'm unbothered.

However, he keeps asking to speak to my mom.

I'm going to tell her what a little whore you are, Suzanne.

I want to tell her what a slut her daughter is.

She would expect it out of Sarah but not out of you.

I'm going to tell her that you let – fuck you in your weird pussy.

She has no idea what her child is up to.

This, as I'm sure you all have recognized, is abusive and

just outright weird on several levels. I may have harassed exes on social media, but it was more of *why aren't you responding to me?* and other desperate behaviors.

First of all, I don't know why he's calling me a whore. I didn't cheat on him or even dare speak to a male gas station attendant the entire two months we dated *or whatever we were doing*. Second of all, who cares if I was a whore? I had the right to do whatever I wanted to before he magically reappeared after my cancer diagnosis. Third of all, how dare he talk about my sister like that?

How. Dare. He?

Fourth of all, here we go with the body shaming again. I don't care what my vagina looks like; everyone's looks different, and that is fucking okay, man.

Get over it.

Naturally, I've already taken care of this. While my mom was sleeping, I created a contact in her phone with his name and number and blocked it. Even if he tried to call, he would never get through. I also used her phone to get into her Facebook account and blocked Dave on both Messenger and the regular Facebook app.

I knew my mom wouldn't mind, but it would take her an hour to do what took me three minutes. I don't want to involve her further with this drama. She has enough to worry about with her health and my dad's inability to work the television.

Jenifer Childers Samples is busy enough.

I did not, for the record, view any of her messages or notifications.

An hour later, my sister wakes up and stumbles out of her old bedroom, pink hair going in three different directions but still looking stylish.

Hey, I have some magic mushrooms if you want to try them later. They have been proven to help with brain cancer.

I think you're referring to micro-dosing, but sure. Why the hell not?

Once Sarah smokes a few cigs, or *walks the dogs*, as she tells my parents, we set up The Samples Sisters' Situation Room in the bedroom aka The Americana Room. We have my laptop, five cell phones, and a bunch of papers (that have nothing to do with anything but my student loans) spread out before us. We can see Dave's old little red house as we make our deviant plans.

1. Sign up for a $29.95 paid background checking service, the same one used by Nev and Max on the show *Catfish*. Since Dave refused to give me his address to send him a card, we will find it this way. What are we going to do?
2. Once we have the address, have a service mail him a free sample of adult diapers because he is a giant baby.
3. Sign me up for a Tinder account because I'm for real done with this bullshit and ready to find the actual love of my life.
4. Keep the background checking service because it will come in very useful for Tinder purposes.

The background check alerts us Dave has roommates. Interesting. He never mentioned them to me. One is female. Of course, this could be faulty information, and naturally, female roommates can be just that: female roommates. However, can you imagine his reaction if I had a male roommate? I'm sure that male roommate would have been fucking my weird pussy within minutes of Dave making that discovery, even if the roommate and I were strictly platonic.

5. Use Sarah's actual phone to pretend to be our mother. Though she has lived in NYC for years, Sarah never got rid of her WV number. Dave doesn't know Sarah or our mom's cell, so this will be easy. We wouldn't even need one of the three burner phones. Even if Dave did think to background check the number, which he wouldn't, it would be easy to explain how they were both on the same family plan. And actually, they were. We wouldn't even have to lie about that.

I'm making a Gas 'N Goods run, Sarah says. *I'll be back with coffee, sugar free Red Bulls, candy, and cigs. This mothafucka is goin' down!*

Although the gas station is about thirty seconds from our house, I know this will likely take her over an hour. Why? Who knows? As my mom always says, *It's better not to sometimes with Sarah.* I take a shower and for the first time in a week, my tears don't intermingle with the DuPont-tainted water. Because the doublewide's walls are so thin, crying in my bedroom or The Americana Room does not provide a safe space for bawling it out. But now, now that Sarah is here, now that we are all back together and none of us have what my dad calls The Covis, now that I have had time to ruminate on my boring MRI results, now that I have rid myself of over 20 years of disgusting grooming and predatory behavior, I feel as free as my sister's dogs do when they run around a big house, pissing in whatever corners they desire.

When Sarah returns, I am in the Samples Sisters' Situation Room in a towel.

Jesus, can you put some clothes on?

I forgot someone else was here.

Sorry, I forgot I had to share this area.

86

She throws a Red Bull at my bare leg, and the cold wakes me up even more to what we are about to do.

Well, get some shit on, we need to get to work!

I sneak into my room so no cat's escape. I want them to run free so badly, and I don't quite understand what my parents think Princess Peppermint might do to them. Sure, she's old and mean, but Delilah might learn one difficult lesson, and that's all she would need.

Okay, I say, breathing hard. Is it the extra weight? The cancer? No, it's just nerves. *What do I do?*

I picked up Mom's phone on the way. She tosses me the giant iPhone, and I somehow catch it. *Unblock him from her account, pretend to be Mom, and say you're tired of your daughters being so out of control and sexually promiscuous. Then ask for his number and say you want to talk to him about it.*

I start giggling like we are middle schoolers again, prank calling boys we pretend we don't like.

Sent!

Dave promptly responds. He has been waiting. Naturally, I think of how he stonewalled me after I got my MRI and made me wait forever to talk to him, and this just makes me want to irritate him that much harder.

I'm glad you understand me, Jenifer, he writes, and then attaches his phone number. We already have it, but it's all part of the game.

Sarah and I wait a few minutes to throw him off.

Hold on, I say.

Hold on! Sarah echoes. This was her catch phrase in adolescence. She was always the last one at the table for dinner, in the car for school or a trip, or anywhere she needed to be.

I'm already laughing.

What are we going to say?

You'll see.

Sarah looks at the message on our mom's phone to get the number and then dials it from her own. She puts the phone on speaker. Dave urgently answers in a huffed tone. *Jenifer? I'm so glad you called. We need to talk about some things.*

Sarah raises her eyebrows and makes the shush symbol with her lips and finger.

Silence.

Dave clears his throat.

Jenifer?

Jenifer, are you there?

We really need to talk, Jenifer, like right now.

Sarah and I sit and stare at one another.

We smirk and try not to laugh.

She counts the seconds on her fingers.

One. Two. Three. Four. Five. Six.

Jenifer! I can't hear you. We need to discuss things your daughter Suzanne has done. You have no idea what a whore she is. I know you didn't raise her to be like that. You won't believe the things she's been doing with men. It's disgusting.

Seven. Eight.

Jenifer?

Nine.

He hangs up.

We burst into laughter.

Stop, Sarah instructs. *Pull it together. We aren't done.*

I listen to her for once.

Ten. Eleven.

Sarah calls back.

We say nothing.

Jenifer, I'm so glad you called back. What I need to tell you is Suzanne has been letting —

fuck her. Black men. I'm trying to stop this behavior, but she won't quit. She is a goddamn whore, Jenifer! I hope you are listening to me because she sure isn't. I'm trying to help her out, but it's impossible.

Twelve. Thirteen.

Jenifer?

Fourteen.

Jenifer?

When Sarah ends the call, she holds up a third phone; she's recorded his entire racist, slut-shaming tirade.

We've done it.

We've fucking fooled the man who thought he was the master.

Am I going to do anything with this? No. I just wanted proof of his bad behavior. Dave always manipulated each situation so carefully; except for one text that could raise the eyebrows of a few cops, he always doled out his verbal abuse over the phone. Most of the time, I was sitting alone in my Boone apartment or far enough away from my parents that no one could hear his constant calumnious behavior.

He thought this was foolproof until my sister got involved.

Now we had him right where we want him.

It's too bad the shit hit the fan before the free diapers arrived.

Harrisville, West Virginia

When I notice the absent feeling in my left hand, I think:

1. Carpal Tunnel
2. I'm on my cell phone way too much
3. No no no no nooooooo no no no

Option c. cannot be right; I am overthinking this. I have

lived with my parents for just a couple of months now, and I am doing well.

As well as any woman in her late 30s can be when living with her parents in the middle of nowhere during a global pandemic.

I confess: I had a weak moment on Father's Day and sent Dave an email.

Hey, hope you had a Happy Father's Day.

I don't know why I did this. I'm sure a psychiatrist would explain these eight words away as a *trauma bond* or something of the sort, but the truth is, I just don't know. I shouldn't have done it, but I did, and I regret it.

But anyway.

I am worried about my hand, but I don't really have much time for that.

I am on a quest.

I need to lose this extra weight, and now is the time. After I drive my mom to physical therapy and pick up my dad's fast food, I have a ton of free hours in the day. Although West Virginia has a reputation for rolling hills, the town of Harrisville is flat enough for someone like me, a former hemiplegic, to practice my newfound walking skills without causing myself further harm. If I do fall, I am confident someone will help me.

No matter how much I don't want to live here forever or how much I resent growing up here, you won't find better people than in Harrisville, West Virginia.

I start small.

Half a mile.

I am worried because I seem to be hallucinating.

Half a mile two days a week.

Small bugs.

Half a mile two days a week in the rain.

Shadow figures.

(Summer equals rain in Harrisville, known fact. One summer we lost power every day, so Sarah and I and played an endless game of Monopoly and other various competitions we made up, including "Who Can Meow the Loudest" and "How Long Can Suzanne Hold Sarah Up in an Airplane Position with her Feet?" Over five minutes, if you're curious.)

Soon enough, I get bored.

Perhaps I think too much of myself.

Perhaps I am reaching a bit.

Perhaps I am overconfident.

Nothing new, I suppose.

Cairo[17]/Cornwallis, West Virginia, Bonds Creek Tunnel, #13, 352 ft.

As my sister sleeps, I head to North Bend State Park, the place where we went for nearly all of our class trips. As a kid, I thought these trips were shit. Why didn't they take us on a bus to the movies? Sure, that would be a two-hour trip and cost way more money, but couldn't the Ritchie County School system manage that? Instead, they took us on these muddy hiking trails and let us prowl around like feral wolf cubs.

Only now do I appreciate those excursions.

The gravelly trail I choose seems unfamiliar; I guess it's been over 20 years since I've traveled these paths with my high school friends when we were goofing off before marching band practice. These particular walkways were once railroad tracks, and occasionally, you can still find old spikes along the path. Trains started moving along the tracks in the mid-1800s and continued until the 1980s; this historical shit bored me as a kid, but as much as I hate to admit it, I am now fascinated and won't leave my retired history teacher father alone.

I have not forgotten about the tunnels.

Somewhere between unique tourist attractions and historical markers, casual hikers can now stroll or bike through the former train tunnels. Number 13, the most obvious on the trail, is naturally crazy popular during Halloween, especially because of a wreck that adds even more mystique. In 1956, a deadly crash occurred in Tunnel #13, killing an engineer and a fireman. Many others were injured. Although another train passed through unscathed just moments earlier, a rockslide hastily devastated the railroad tracks in the fateful moments between the first and second engines.

Unable to stop, the second vehicle exploded into the rockslide and tumbled out of the egress, off of a bridge, and into a creek.

The tunnel itself, though? Not scary at all. At 353 feet, you don't need a headlamp or flashlight to get through this bad boy.

Even for a disabled person like myself, #13 feels like walking through a slightly dark hallway. I can do this. I feel good, refreshed, like a new person after walking through. I feel proud of myself for accomplishing this walk. Others may have crashed and died here, but I have made it my bitch.

Who needs a girlfriend or boyfriend when I have tunnels to keep me company?

I don't know how many tunnels exist yet, but I know I need to find them all before I go.

PART II
WILD & WONDERFUL

Point Pleasant, West Virginia

You aren't a true West Virginia Gen X/Millennial (or Millennium, as my mom says) unless you have a picture with the Mothman statue in Point Pleasant, West Virginia.

Because we can't think of anything better to do, Sarah and I mask up and make the two-hour drive. This excursion feels eerily similar to when she drove me to radiation; despite the cool spring WV air, the windows of my tiny Scion must be down the entire time so she can blow her ashes into the backseat, which doubles as the trunk.

My favorite picture is of me, my back to the camera, reaching toward The Mothman in an arc of praise.

Harrisville, West Virginia

Before my sister leaves, she helps me create a Tinder account.

You need a distraction, she says.

I have enough distractions, I tell her.

*You need a **fun** distraction*, she answers, and then she is off to Texas before I can delete the app.

I have no idea what the fuck I am doing.

I mean, I know how to swipe right and left. Beyond that, I am lost.

If you are married or have been in a long-term relationship (gay, straight, or somewhere in-between), you might find yourself wondering at times, what else is out there? Am I missing out? Is everyone having fun except for me? Maybe there's something better?

I am here to tell you—unless you are in an abusive or toxic relationship requiring you to flee, boring is good. Stay where you are. Water that grass, instead of seeing what's greener on the other side.

I text my sister late one night: *Okay, I thought everyone on Tinder was looking for a relationship.*

Haaaaa yeah, I thought that for about ten minutes too when I first got on there.

I have seen every single episode of the show *Catfish*. I consider myself intuitive and able to read people relatively well. I have dated good people, shitty people, and people everywhere in the middle.

But Tinder?

Tinder is the brain cancer of dating.

As one might imagine, the queer scene in extremely rural West Virginia is not exactly thriving. This isn't to say it doesn't exist, but for someone who has been gone for over 20 years, I don't know exactly where to look.

I'm also not sure I want to.

Or maybe I do.

I just want a stable relationship with someone who respects me.

Why I thought I could find this on Tinder is a self-help book I don't have time to write.

I toggle my settings to both men and women, but only two women emerge in the swiping game.

A social justice warrior named Avery, who obviously just wants to be pen pals, and a lesbian with a lip ring named Deb, who won't leave me alone for two minutes.

Cisgender men on Tinder are boldly horrible and ask three questions right away:

1. Do you like anal?
2. Do you hookup?
3. Are you shaved?

The clever ones wait a couple of conversations before getting to these very important interrogations, but some matches just ask them outright. *It's a match! Do you like anal? Do you hookup? Are you shaved?*

Un. Match.

I heard about what a shitshow Tinder was but let me tell you: Unless you are a woman talking to men, no matter your sexual orientation, you have no idea how dark and dangerous this dating tunnel is. At times, I wonder if I'll ever emerge.

To navigate online dating, I turn to the internet to learn a new vocabulary.

Sarah also helps me out by warning me about the ***roster, n.*: the handful of people, definitely ranked, though this ranking can change, you talk to, text, call, or see throughout the week.**

Because we are in the middle of a pandemic, THE pandemic, thus far I'm only texting and occasionally Facetiming or calling people. Then, you have to realize these people on your roster definitely have their own roster, and where do you fall? If James is your number one but you're his number three, what's going to happen?

I am not here to confuse anyone.

Still acutely aware I could perish in a matter of months, I decide to be open about my brain cancer. For my bio, I write a long paragraph about being an online English professor, an author, loving cats, looking for a serious relationship, and having glioblastoma. On Tinder, I ramble on and on until the app tells me I can't type anything else.

I don't know why I do this.

I suppose I don't want anyone to think I am going to go water skiing with them when the time comes. Or rock climbing. Or BASE jumping off the New River Gorge Bridge, though I wish I could.

My initial roster includes[1]:

1. Marcus the Mechanic, a ginger fellow from Ohio.
2. Tim the Attorney, an indie music afficionado from Charleston, WV.
3. Damien who works in "Travel" from somewhere in Ohio?

Notes on Marcus the Mechanic:

- Background check comes back clean.
- Answers texts quickly but not stalkerish.
- Doesn't have a thick accent, although he is from rural Ohio. I wouldn't be turned off if he did, but I find it fascinating he doesn't.
- Noted on his profile he was "looking for the Kelly to his Ryan," which piques my interest as an *Office*

fan. Doesn't take the typical "looking for the Pam to my Jim" route.

- Always wants to FaceTime; I'm not much into FaceTiming, but it's nice he shows effort.
- Asked me to float down a river with him and his friends. Although this sounds like fun, I have to decline because I can no longer swim. I haven't EXPLAINED THE THING yet, so I just simply text back, I can't swim. Sad face. He says okay and starts talking about something else.

He takes the news of my cancer well; although I don't currently have any tumors and I'm not in treatment, I tell him how *glioblastoma doesn't really go away.* He basically says, *Okay, I understand,* and then says he will tell me one of his own secrets.

This feels like a safe exchange of information, like protected emotional intercourse.

Okay, deep breath, Marcus texts.

I find myself also taking a deep breath. What is he going to text me? Does he have nine kids? Is he still married? It's got to be an STD. That's fine; we can work around that. Maybe he accidentally killed someone. I rode with a rideshare driver once who confessed he accidentally murdered a road patcher because it was dark, and he wasn't paying attention. Your guess is as good as mine as to how he was hired as a professional driver.

I don't make these judgments.

I got drunk with my parents a few years ago, and when I woke up, my dad was giving me a blowjob.

I am shocked. That's a horrific secret to share, and although I don't know him, I immediately want to give Marcus a hug. I can't believe anyone would do that to a kid.

99

Oh my god. I'm so sorry. I don't know what to say.

It's okay. I haven't seen or spoken to them since then.

That's horrible. Obviously, that should never happen to anyone. I can't believe that.

I don't ever see them anymore. I wish I had the type of relationship you have with your family. It's just unfortunate.

I don't text back for a few minutes, not because I want to avoid him but because I can't believe how terrible some people in the world are. No matter how angry I get with my parents, I am lucky to have them and grateful I can come home whenever I want with no questions asked. People in Marcus' situation can't do that.

Yes, I'm very fortunate, I text. *I am so sorry that happened to you. I'll be honest, I don't really know what to say, other than that's fucking horrible.*

I don't know what to say about your cancer, other than it's also horrible! he responds, and I laugh for the first time in a long time.

Maybe this online dating thing isn't so bad.

Cornwallis, West Virginia, Tunnel #12, 577 ft.²

However, I'm obviously not the type to sit at home all summer and message people from Tinder. My online semester wraps up, and I have tunnels to find. I know they are out there; at this point, I don't know how many, but I'm willing to go on a blind search to find out.

Just past Tunnel #13 is Tunnel #12, or The Nameless as Far as I Know tunnel. Although it's close to #13, this one seems forgotten.

Dark.

Decrepit.

Lost.

At 577 feet, #12 is longer than #13 and seems like an endless shunt of black space. I don't have a flashlight or head-lamp, but I say *fuck it* and take my chances.

Once I am out of the light and can only hear the dripping water, I lose myself in the darkness.

Falling is the only option.

The best choice.

The only way to escape this quagmire.

I don't want to ruin my sweatpants, but it's just mud and possibly animal dung.

I cannot survive forever in Tunnel #12.

I feel like a spirit.

My cellphone flashlight is nothing more than a pinprick beam. Is this how my brain looked to my surgeon? How much could he see? I tried to watch craniotomies on YouTube, but I couldn't get past the initial incision.

I did not have the stomach.

After a single semester off work, I returned to teaching. Sure, I still had to complete chemo and had physical, occupa-tional, and speech therapy, but I needed money. As a solo woman, I couldn't sit in my apartment until I died.

When I fall in Tunnel #12, I forget to protect my hands. I had collapsed before on these trails a few days ago, and the results were heinous. I picked pebbles out of my palms for weeks and nursed an infected knee. A truck nearly ran me over. Did they see me and not care? I'm not sure. I rolled into a ditch and didn't move until the vehicle sped away.

And when I could no longer hear the motor, I told myself *in through your nose and out through your mouth. You just have to breathe.*

I did not want to become another casualty of these trails, of these tunnels.

I had improved my strength and mobility, and now I could

slump to the ground in this cavernous darkness and still make my way out of here on my own.

I am not sure if my palms land in equine shit or mud. Many people ride horses through the tunnels, but they are told to dismount before entering. Too often, the horses get spooked and toss the riders.

Once my knees hit the earth, I finally exhale. I roll to my ass and listen to the lonely drops of water splash into puddles. I remove my hood so I might feel less dizzy, but nothing helps. I am engulfed by these endless shadows and have no idea which direction is out. I no longer care about the mess on my sweatpants; I just want to sit here and feel less lightheaded.

Visit me, ghosts, I taunt. *Come and find me.* I've always believed in the paranormal. There's far too much out there we just don't know. At this point, I would welcome an apparition. Perhaps a vision would shepherd me out of here. *If you don't want to leave, at least guide me toward some light.*

My voice eerily echoes.

As if I am a cavewoman looking to the walls for a story, I suddenly hallucinate petroglyphs forming before me.

A woman smiles with her friends, all of them at the ballet barre in first position. In the next iteration, a woman stands in front of people seated at writing desks. Finally, the same woman sits at a table with two cats and a dog at her feet.

The right foot is twisted and limp, like a disinterested lover.

As I stare at the story in stone, the drawing of the woman elevates from the tunnel wall and shifts into a pale silhouette. Her friends stay engraved, but she lifts from the markings and resembles a shape made from fancy cigarette smoke. She morphs into a fully fleshed human and stares back at me with passionate intensity.

I recognize this bright smile she gives me *before everything happened.*

I recognize the way she shakes, the way her eyes refuse to blink when the surgeon says *unfortunately*.

I recognize the look of horror when she pulls hair from its roots and holds balls of brunette strands in her small hands.

And then, as if I am waking from a nightmare, the woman disappears like thin whisps of smoke from a locomotion long gone.

Harrisville, West Virginia

Back safely at home, I ask myself: Why stop with Marcus?

I am enjoying the attention I'm getting from Tinder.

In high school, the only reason boys talked to me was because I was smart and could help them get good grades in class. College? I was mostly an introvert. I had one boyfriend, but he annoyed me, and I was never really attracted to him. There had been other boyfriends and girlfriends scattered throughout, but this. This! This was the perfect kind of attention for me. I could post a few pictures and text people all day long. I didn't have to meet up with them unless I really wanted to, and I could just explore tunnels in the afternoons and respond when I felt like it.

Online dating was meant for people like me.

The attention never ends. What do I owe these people? Nothing.

I get bored and feel empty with this, though.

I am not the type of person to mess with people's heads.

It's fun for a minute, but I can't keep it up.

It's a lot of *Hey, what are you up to?*

Them: *Nothing, just work.*

Me: *Oh, cool! I just found another abandoned train tunnel in my quest, and then I'm planning my summer courses for school. I'm also going to listen to some new music tonight. What type of music do you like?*

Okay, maybe I'm a bit intense sometimes, but I'm doing everything I can to distract from the real mess inside my brain.

No response.

I get back on Tinder to swipe more.

Left left left—is that a guy in black face? Jesus H. Christ. No, it's a coal miner. Okay. Pshew. —left left left right sure why not right left right.

It's a match!

Do I even want to match with this person?

I close Tinder.

B. has sent you a message.

I open Tinder back up.

Okay, hear me out. B. lives in Parkersburg and has long hair he wears in a ponytail. He's not ugly but he lives in Parkersburg. Eh. Whatever. I'm in need of conversation. *The cops are all bastards, and I have made this design to demonstrate how terrible they are.* He sends me a screenshot of a mandala he sketched with a blue colored pencil. I don't see anything special about this mandala or how it relates to what's going on in the world right now, but I play along. *Love it! Did you make it?* I mean, I'm all for creativity, even if the mandala looks like a third grader drew it. *Yes, I did! I'm so glad you get it! This is what West Virginia is about to look like in two months when the aliens come and take all the cops back to ouder space.*

Ouder space.

Wow, I write. *Go on. I'm intrigued.*

Yeah, so the aliens will be back sooner rather than later and they are taking the bad guys with them. This is enough! I have something else to show you.

I prepare myself for the ever-unwanted dick pic.

It's another mandala, this time in red.

How does this one makes you feel?

Oooh, not good at all.

I guess I was supposed to feel good about the red mandala as well because Parkersburg Ponytail unmatches me.

Oh well. What's Tinder if not a night of bizarre conversation?

If the aliens ever came back to Parkersburg, I never heard about it from him.

Maybe he was Indrid Cold.

I'll never know for sure.

Cairo/Cornwallis, West Virginia, Tunnels #13 (Bonds Creek Tunnel) & #12

These tunnels become my solace, my obsession.

I feel oddly secure in the solitary darkness and free to let my mind wander back to when these railways were active. It's difficult to believe a place so tranquil, quiet, and lonesome, except for the occasional trail birdwatcher, once bustled with activity and industry. My grandfather, originally from the Louisville, KY, area, met my grandmother while working on a railway and staying at her family's now-demolished Whitehall Hotel in Harrisville.

I'm not terribly interested in the love stories, though.

I'm more interested in the darkness.

When I'm not falling and getting gravel lodged underneath my skin, I like sitting in the carved-out, crumbling lantern embrasures and listening to the water drip by my feet like a distant fever dream of a past life.

Though it's late spring and warming toward summer, I still wear my winter boots. My friends Kate and Steve sent me a pair of headlamps so I don't fuck myself up too badly in the murkiness. There's obviously no cell service in these beasts, and I don't have to answer to anyone about what I'm picking up for *supper*, what exactly I'm doing back in Harrisville, West Virginia, if I'm shaved or if I like to hookup, or what stage my cancer is in now.

I can just exist.

I can be.

I can wonder what the hell happened when a lantern kid accidentally stepped off one of these embrasures at the wrong time and the train couldn't stop.

I bet this happened more than anyone ever admitted, and I am suspicious that no one kept track of such a thing, though I obviously have no proof of any of this.

At first, I don't think of finding all 13 remaining tunnels on the North Bend Rail Trail; I simply view this as an opportunity to improve my walking and get out of the house. Sure, I am able to walk about two miles a day now on flat ground but so what? How can I actually be good at walking if I can't do it in a tunnel as cavernous as my own brain, stumbling around in there like a novice neurosurgeon who doesn't quite know how to resect tumors correctly yet? I like digging into the discovery, the unknown, the creepiness of it all. Especially during the day, I don't see a soul out here. When I do fall, I don't have to feel embarrassed or ashamed or less than anyone or anything.

Number 12 quickly becomes my favorite; I always slip or completely fall at least once when I'm trudging through the blackness. I also feel sorry for this tunnel because she is terribly neglected and perhaps on the verge of collapse at some point in the near future. As far as I know, this tunnel does not have a name or any donor, and honestly, after being abandoned and abused by lovers and people I thought were my closest friends, I feel the same way.

Same way, #12.

Same.

I sigh when I see the sunlight on the other end, though. What would happen if I didn't make it through? Would it, could it, be worse than perishing from brain cancer? A part of me doesn't think so. I could just freeze to death between her trestles, in this dark womb. I would finally feel protected.

I would finally feel safe, no matter how badly it hurt.

Harrisville, West Virginia

Attorney Tim intrigues me.

When I ask him if he likes certain bands, he always texts back the name of a song and says things like, *"Chicago"! That's my jam!* and when I text him indie tracks and videos, he says he watches and likes them. Being into the same music isn't a requirement for me, but this makes me feel like we have stuff in common.

You should look up a band called The Good Life, I tell him. *The lead singer has the same name as you!*

He sure does! Tim says.

I smile.

He already drops the l-word when I send him selfies.

I love that.

Love that shirt on you.

You should pull it down a bit.

At first, I don't. Why would I? I don't know this man, and all we have done is text. But then the *Good morning!* texts start coming through, and the messages show no sign of stopping throughout the day.

The more we text, the more interested I become.

What attorney has time to text throughout the day like this? I don't have a summer class until the second session, so I have all the hours in the universe, but why does he have so much time? He is either lying, terrible at his job, or absolutely so stellar a lawyer, he has a ton of free moments.

One problem.

His number shows absolutely nothing on the background check.

This has not happened before, so I don't know what to make of it.

Unfortunately, I like it.

I don't know Tim's last name, but I've seen enough episodes of *Catfish* to handle this, I think.

He's got to be real, but something still seems off.

Tim responds so quickly, it's hard to avoid becoming infatuated with the attention. He wants to know everything about me. He lets me talk about myself, and for once, I find it easy to do so. I try to hold back, but I've let so much of myself become consumed with other people lately—Dave, CK, my parents—it feels rather nice to have someone only want to know about me.

At first, I don't consider it strange that he never tells me about himself.

Of course, I ask questions, but he rarely elaborates.

He has twin daughters and a dog. I don't ask for a picture of the daughters because that would be super weird and intrusive, but I do ask for a snapshot of the pup. Although I'm far more interested in him than I have been in anyone else, something about Tim puts me on guard, and I want as much evidence as I can gather when I inevitably present it to Emily and her younger sister Cathleen, who knows way more about online dating and the internet than either of us.

His dog, Burt, is a handsome raven-colored boy with a goofy grin.

If this pic was culled from the web, it should be easy to find.

. . .

Pennsboro, WV, Cunningham's Tunnel, #8, 588 ft.

There you are, I say to Tunnel #8 when I turn around and spot her wide mouth, open and ready to welcome me.

Like my mother I have a terrible sense of direction and get lost as easily as a ghost trapped in the wrong time period.

I walked exactly three miles down the North Bend Rail Trail, thinking I was following the correct direction of a GPS location to find #8, when I realized the tunnel was not there. I didn't even know if I was on the correct section of trail. I lost cell service two miles ago, and I hadn't even looked when I did have service to make certain I was on the correct path.

After trudging the three miles back to the car, I feel defeated and tired. I don't know if I can find the tunnel today.

I get out of the car, turn around, and walk about fifty feet.

The tunnel is right in front of me.

Dammit.

I needed the exercise anyway.

I never spent much time in Pennsboro, another small town[3] about a thirteen-minute drive from our house. This is no excuse for me to completely turn the wrong way and miss a giant, abandoned train tunnel right in front of me, but perhaps I can blame the brain cancer.

Is it back? Is it causing me to miss giant stone structures right in front of the trailhead? Is this what happens right before I die? Am I already dead? People speak of the white light—is it really just a black hole in the form of a giant train tunnel?

Calm down, Suzanne.

I have a much scarier, urgent problem.

I need to take a shit.

There are no bathrooms along this section of the Rail Trail. Although I've certainly danced off into the woods before to pee, that was an earlier time when I felt more confident regarding my mobility and balance. Lately, and I don't know if it's because I've gotten older or because my body changed after what I've been through, I have not been processing lactose well.

I need to go now.

Although I'm alone, anyone could show up on the trail at whatever moment; they appear like specters, these hikers. I'm so slow, I would never be able to shit beside of the trail before someone would see me.

I don't really have time to think.

Tunnel #8— she is dark.

At 588 feet, I could get away with it.

No, Suzanne, you cannot.

The horses do it all the time.

People around here love the Rail Trail for horse riding, and I don't blame them.

Also, there is horse shit everrrrrrrrywhere, which always makes for interesting falls inside the tunnel. Is it mud? Is it horse shit? Who knows!

My point: Would people shit matter?

I don't have time.

I have to do this.

No.

These tunnels have become sacred to me. My place to relearn walking properly, my place to relearn myself.

How could I fuck up somewhere I love so much?

I don't have a choice.

I walk to the middle of the tunnel and click my headlamp off. Thank the Fogwoman this is a curved tunnel; I would have at least a few seconds to pull my pants up before bikers or hikers would appear in the darkness and see me.

I make sure I am as far from the middle of the tunnel as possible and relieve a horse load of my own shit. Something about being in the hospital for a month makes actions like this so much easier. Once you've had three CNAs, male and female, help you take a dump after brain surgery and then one announces *I think you got your period*, all decorum disappears.

I finish my business and pull up my sweatpants.

I always take a couple photos of both tunnel ends, so I quickly exit and snap what I need and get back in the car.

I'm sorry, Tunnel #8.

At my worst, I am a horse.

Parkersburg, West Virginia

Parkiesburg.

That's what the old fellows in the Mid-Ohio Valley call it, just as my grandfather did before he died.

To do anything in my hometown, you have to drive the forty minutes to Parkersburg. You may recognize the town's name from the following:

1. Again, home of the DuPont chemical plant, responsible for dumping PFAS[4] into the Ohio River and contaminating thousands of animals and people, likely giving them cancer.
2. Hometown of Patsy Ramsey, pageant queen and mother of JonBenét Ramsey.

But for the people of Harrisville, Parkersburg is where you go to see a movie or simply get stuff done.

Today, I must brave the DMV. I have tried multiple times to get my car tags updated, but much to my father's chagrin, I have failed.

There's always something.

This time, I actually get my license, but for the tags, the lady tells me *you gotta go to Fast Eddie's, hon.*

Fast Eddie's?

This can't be a real place.

If it's a real place, Fast Eddie's certainly can't be a legitimate business to get updated car tags. I follow the directions anyway and find Fast Eddie's hidden behind some other business' staircase. They ask me to sit in a broken chair, and I am worried the seat will fall apart completely and send me tumbling to the floor, where, I am convinced, the coronavirus thrives. A broken air-conditioning unit hangs from the window like a loose tooth.

Instead, the lady at Fast Eddie's just screams at me from her desk.

Whatcha here for?

I need to get updated car tags.

Do you have your title?

No—the car isn't paid off yet, but they said that you could—

Can't do nothing bout that one.

She pulls out a Lucky Strike from her leather purse. I can tell it's an extension of her long, gnarly finger. I wonder if I have somehow drifted back to 1985. I think she might light the cig right then and there, but she waits.

I'm frustrated. This is my third time coming to Parkiesburg to get this shit dealt with, and I just keep (illegally) driving in circles. Mr. Samples will not be happy about this, not at all. At least I will bring my parents home Olive Garden. My dad has a current obsession with their tiramisu, or what he calls *good cake.*

What am I supposed to do then? My bank won't release the official title, and no one will let me update my tags without the official title.

Sorry, she says, tapping the Lucky Strike on the desk. The air-conditioner I thought was broken suddenly pops on, making me nearly fall out of the seat. *Don't know what to tell ya.*

I wonder if I can gamble a few bucks here at Fast Eddie's so it's not a wasted trip.

Fast Edwina is out the door before I can stand from the broken chair.

When I get back to the car, I feel like I just lost a million bucks in a slot machine.

I check my phone: three texts from Marcus the Mechanic.

9:41: Good morning!

10:43: How are you today?

1:53: Guess I'm not getting a text back then.

Something about this irritates the fuck out of me. Marcus the Mechanic and I have never met, and I'm under no obligation to text him every single hour of every single day.

I am not his girlfriend.

I am no one's girlfriend.

I only belong to me.

I started using Tinder to boost myself esteem, help myself heal from a controlling relationship, and hopefully meet someone nice.

Not this passive-aggressive bullshit.

Nope.

Hey, sorry! I was at the DMV all day.

I stay polite.

He's been through a lot.

Cairo, West Virginia, The Silver Run Tunnel, #19, 1376 ft.

I've put off exploring The Silver Run Tunnel for quite some time.

It's the most well-known and obsessed over tunnel, and

probably overrated. Nonetheless, I need to see the haunted train tunnel for myself.

Sadly, the tunnel itself seems to be a ghost.

I cannot find it anywhere.

Only about nine miles from Harrisville, my dad assures me I will be able to locate this tunnel no problem. He's taken multiple classes there on field trips, and it's not too far from a trailhead big enough to park a bus. I could search the internet for GPS coordinates, but I consider that cheating, and I never have cell service outside of an internet connection in these towns.

I slide the barn door open to my parents' side of the new house, which we finally moved into a few days ago.

My dad stands beside of the fridge with a cold slice of pizza, his belt the only reason his pants cling to his nearly nonexistent hips.

Morning, Suzanne. Want some pizza?

I realize with startling clarity: I too stand beside the fridge in the morning and eat cold pizza.

Dammit.

No thank you. I'm off to find the Silver Run Tunnel.

Mr. Samples looks excited. He taught at Cairo Middle School for years, and I know this was his favorite school.

Easy to find, my dad says. *It's near the school. Just don't let aliens abduct you or something.*

I look at him with confusion. I know one of his brothers claimed an alien abduction once, but I'm not sure I understand why aliens might snatch me near an abandoned train tunnel in Cairo, West Virginia, though now that I'm thinking of it, it just might be the perfect place.

The problem: I cannot find the tunnel from the trailhead in Cairo.

The problem: None of these tunnels are really that easy to find.

The problem: I have a horrible sense of direction.

Although I don't realize where I'm headed, I just start walking toward Ellenboro and eventually find #19, the Silver Run Tunnel.

At first glance, I don't see why this is supposed to be the THE HAUNTED TUNNEL, though it's easy to see people clearly believe it is: So far, #19 is the only tunnel I've seen with graffiti. People have painted the walls with little ghosties to frighten the children. Once inside the tunnel, however, I see the allure.

The sun really didn't come out today, but outside of the tunnel, there isn't rain or any sort of precipitation. Inside the tunnel, however, a thick white cloud rests in the middle like a funeral fog.

I haven't seen this in any of the other tunnels.

I don't feel scared I don't feel scared I don't feel scared.

I've never done this before, but I decide to sit in one of the safety alcoves and chill for a minute.

I think of this tunnel's heroine.

It's a typical urban legend.

The version I've heard, though I'm sure others exist, is a stunning black-haired bride boarded the train with her new husband. Despite her allure, her bridegroom had a mistress he preferred.

Here's where the story, like many tales, becomes a bit blurred and obfuscated.

The new bride, still in her white wedding gown and with her husband on their way to the honeymoon, either:

1. discovered her husband's infidelity and, incredibly distraught, stepped off the train in Tunnel #19 to her death.

2. was pushed by her new husband off the train into Tunnel #19 to her demise so he could be with the mistress shame free.

Look, either way, it was the fuckboy's fault.

Now the Lady in White haunts the tunnel and a constant layer of fog serves as her home.

Nothing about this tunnel frightens me, though.

Instead of being fearful of #19, I feel oddly at home here. I sit in one of the embrasures and listen to the water drip and echo like a faucet in an abandoned home. It's soaking wet, but I don't care. I pop off my headlamp and decide to hang here for a few minutes.

I have this odd feeling no one else will be here today, except for what remains unseen.

I might be out of my fucking mind, but I start communicating with the Lady in White.

So here we are, right in the middle of a global pandemic, I tell her, not expecting an answer.

Drip drip drip.

Okay, so you're here. Very cool. Anyway, I have this brain cancer problem. I don't know how much longer I'm going to live. The cancer is called glioblastoma, and I was supposed to die less than a year after I was diagnosed, but I somehow survived. Can you honestly believe that? Sometimes I can't. I was paralyzed on my right side for a long time, but I ended up working through that, and now my right foot is really the only problem. Anyway, you probably don't care.

Drip drip.

I started trying to date people, and I ended up in a relation-

ship with this girl who straight up idolized me, and I honestly could not live up to what she thought I was. I could never meet her expectations, and she was young and drank a lot, which happens when you're young, but then she got violent when she was drunk, and when things got really bad, she pushed me into a wall, and then she told everyone I was the crazy one.

Drip drip.

And then! Then! I ended up in a relationship with someone I idolized for a long time, and he turned out to be the most verbally abusive person I've ever encountered. My days began with screaming phone calls and ended with stonewalling because he was scanning my Facebook account to see what men "liked" my pictures. Which is just totally ridiculous. I completely lost myself and even deleted my account for a minute just to keep that bastard happy, but I'm sure you can guess exactly what happened.

Drip.

Yep. He just found something else to scream about. And to think—I almost moved to Virginia to be with him. That would have been the biggest mistake of my life, my god.

Drip Drip.

Now I'm trying online dating, and even though it's a scary hellscape out there, it's better than waking up every morning to someone absolutely screaming bloody murder at me for doing nothing wrong.

And this cancer thing. It could come back at any moment. I'm not even supposed to say I'm in remission because I guess the brain cancer cells in glioblastoma never quite go away? It's very confusing. I feel like I'm in remission, so I'm going to say I am, even if I'm not supposed to. Whatever. I have dreams all the time about dying from these damn brain tumors. Even when I'm sleeping, I can't get away from this shit.

In a way, I'm jealous of you. I know that's fucked up.

Drip drip.

Okay, I shouldn't have said that. You were young and someone really screwed you over. But think of it this way—you died before anything could eat you away. That seems fair, right?

Drip.

Yeah, I guess nothing is quite fair, to be honest. I'm sorry.

This is so much better than a therapy session.

I stay seated in the safety alcove and close my eyes.

I hear the train churning down the tracks in the distance.

I feel the fog prickling my skin cold.

I smell the West Virginia coal fueling the engine.

I see the Lady in White standing on the train, her arms barely clinging to the caboose, smiling as the train barrels through the tunnel. She turns her head and gives her new, duplicitous husband a final kiss before letting go of the handles and falling from the train, backbone crumpling into the ribbon rails.

I stand from the embrasure and try to catch her in my arms.

She falls through my embrace, already morphed into a fog, misty and forever free.

Harrisville, West Virginia/Ohio Backroads

Despite the initial yellow flag of being pissy with me for not returning texts on time, I agree to a date with Marcus. He senses I am nervous about my first Tinder encounter, so he offers to pick me up at my parents' house.

In hindsight, this was a terrible idea. At the time, I was thinking about my parents identifying him should I go missing; I wasn't thinking about him having my permanent address. Plus, I had talked to him for about a month-and-a-half now, and he seemed safe enough. He was actually putting in some effort, which anyone on Tinder knows means something.

Everything goes well at first. He picks me up, shakes my parents' hands, and is a perfect gentleman as he helps me into his car. Just as he is on text and Facetime, Marcus is a decent conversationalist. I see no further red or yellow flags, and though a mechanic is not what I would call *my type*, I'm enjoying myself as we drive back to Ohio, which Marcus insists on.

I can't really disagree.

There's nothing to do in Harrisville, and he knows of more options in Ohio. I tell him I won't be going into any restaurants because I'm terrified of Covid, and he complies.

So far, so good.

He chooses Chipotle, brings burritos back to the car, and we pull into a park. The day is rancidly hot, but I pick at my burrito while Marcus regales me with war stories. He charms me with his tale of friendship and love about how his *buddy in Iraq died in the trenches. I fucked up my leg and had to relearn to walk again, just like you did.* He raises his hand and gives me a high five. I feel a sense of sadness for his friend and camaraderie for what we both went through.

Just as I'm deep in my feels and fried rice, I see it.

His penis.

Out in the middle of the daylight, flopping below his steering wheel.

I make eye contact with my burrito as quickly as I can.

Well, there it is.

He says this like he's doing the most normal thing in the world, showing me his dick in public, in the middle of a park, right after telling me about his friend's death and relearning to walk again. I've learned a few things about PTSD symptoms, but flashing people is not one of them.

Well, say something!

I can sense he's getting angry.

I am terrified.

It's great! I say, forcing every bit of enthusiasm I have left in me. He leaves his dick hanging there like a wet cigarette. *But you have to...put it away. We are in public. In daylight. At a park. You...you can't do that. There are children right there.*

He zips his pants up.

Okay, I just thought you would want to see it.

I did not want to see it.

I did not want someone to call the cops.

Well, perhaps I did want someone to call the cops, but I needed a way home.

I did not want to get arrested on a first date.

I return to my burrito; despite seeing what I just saw, I am still hungry.

I need to tell you something, Marcus says.

Great. He's definitely murdered someone and not while in the Army, maybe the last woman he took on a Tinder date. This cannot be good.

I'm just going to say it, he states. *I love you.*

Oh god. This might be worse than him admitting to murder. I could think of a way to respond to that. I've never had someone say they love me on a first date, especially after whipping out their dick in public. I try to get my window down, but he has the child lock on.

I'm fucking panicking.

I need air, no matter how still and humid.

I need help.

I need out of here.

Um, can you fix the window, please?

Yeah, sure, I have it like that for when my son is with me.

You have a son?

This is news to me, though I'm thankful for the subject

change. In two minutes, I've seen a dick I didn't want to see, had a first date say he loved me, and found out about a son.

Let's take a drive, he says.

I would honestly like to go home, but now I am scared and don't want to anger him. He had mentioned a *personality disorder* on FaceTime, but I didn't think much of it at the time. At this point, I've rarely dated someone who didn't have a personality disorder, but now I'm thinking I should have asked more questions as a matter of safety.

Marcus stops at a gas station, I'm assuming to get a pop or candy or something, but he emerges like any good hillbilly with an 18-pack of Keystone and a Diet Coke for me. I appreciate the gesture, but I haven't drunk Diet Coke in decades because I can't stand the taste of aspartame.

I also assume he's going to drop me off back in Harrisville then wait until he gets to his own home to open up the Keystone, but you can probably guess by now, I am also wrong about that.

We aren't even out of the parking lot before he cracks open a Keystone and chugs out of the can like it's a sparkling water.

I am going to die and not of brain cancer.

I can't help myself.

You seriously aren't drinking that and driving, are you?

Oh, it takes way more than this to get me drunk. 'Sides, the cops around here all know me.

Is that supposed to comfort me? I don't feel better.

Twilight blankets over Ohio, and I ask Marcus to take me home.

I thought you'd never ask, he says as he crushes a can with his left fist. Although I usually can't stand Diet Coke, I take giant swigs, partially to calm myself down and partially to please him because I am terrified.

I'm hoping he can get me home and back to his own house before getting wasted. Right now, it's not looking great.

I am worried I am scared I am horrified.

He cracks open another Keystone as he pulls onto some backroads. I am terrible with directions, but I know this is no route to my house.

Home.

He is taking me to his home.

Did I ever tell you I was All-State Choir in high school? Marcus asks. He did tell me he made All-State Choir in 2004, and I felt for him. I can tell he hangs onto that honor, like the high school quarterback from 1989 who can't quit talking about it. He fiddles with his phone as he swivels the car around a turn, and though I'm only drinking Diet Coke, I'm about to vomit. He turns the volume up on a song I don't recognize and sings along with his entire Keystone spirit. He has what my nana would call *a very nice voice*, and he's so in his head, he shuts his eyes.

Marcus!

I can't take it anymore. He's drinking and singing and driving on these roads curvier than I am, and shutting his eyes is the final moment for me. He returns to present-day Ohio from his 2004 fantasy and downs another beer. Marcus keeps belting out the song, but he does keep his eyes open and on the road.

Small victories?

He drives deeper into the woods.

They are going to interview my cousin Amanda on *Dateline*, for sure. We have discussed this; she's the one I want to talk.

Marcus finally slows down and pulls onto a gravel road. I hope he's turning around, but he stops and belches. I spot some wild turkeys on a sagging, lightless porch.

Are we at your house? I ask excitedly. I've had a brief talk with myself and my Diet Coke. Although I have zero acting skills except for that one time I was *Chorus Girl #3* in high school, I am going to act like I love Marcus. I am going to pretend I am having the time of my life. I am going to be excited and interested and give him so much attention that he will be more than thrilled to take me home and get me out of his hair.

We are! I thought I'd show you around before I take you back.

Yessss! I've always wanted a guy to bring me to his house on the first date. I think I love you too!

Hell yeah!

My god. It's working.

Can you help me up the porch? You're super strong, so I know you won't let me fall. I've always wanted a boyfriend like you.

Sure thing, yes.

His house, if I can even call it that, is covered in a thick layer of black mold in most rooms. There's a sheetless mattress on his bedroom floor, and the kitchen linoleum curls up toward the ceiling like rotting wood. He gives me the grand tour as if he's showing me around a mansion instead of a shack. His two pit bulls greet me with wiggly butts, and I see a tortoiseshell kitty peek out from around the dusty fridge. He screams at the pit bulls to *back off* of me, and I desperately want to take the animal's home. I ask if I can use his bathroom. I don't have to, but at this point, it's all writing material.

It does not disappoint.

I've seen one other toilet that looks like this, two others if you count the *Saw* movies. The other belonged to one of my boyfriends in grad school, and the corroded commode was the least of his worries. This toilet has at least five visible bugs and multiple layers of dark filth covering the ceramic. I jiggle the handle, but there is no hope for a flush. The room reeks of stale towels and beer-stained carpet. Marcus' shack doesn't have a bathtub but a standalone shower that looks more like a toilet than the actual commode.

Proof: There is a pile of shit in the left corner.

When I return to the living area, Marcus pats a spot on the lumpy couch (does it have fleas? Certainly, it has fleas) and invites me to sit. I recognize the sounds of an *Office* episode and realize I'm here for at least 22 more minutes.

Play along, Suzanne, play along.

Marcus and I initially connected over our love of *The Office*, and looking back, it was definitely the only thing we had in common and something I could surely find with someone else.

I can't help myself.

I have to say something.

This is a real bachelor pad.

Oh yeah. I live here for free since I'm doing renovations.

Don't laugh don't laugh don't laugh.

Whenever I try to stop myself from laughing, I think about the severity of my situation and how I am wasting my time with clowns like Marcus.

How are the renovations going?

Pretty well, he says. *I'm getting there.*

Don't laugh don't laugh don't laugh.

I can't help myself; I start to laugh, but thankfully, it's timed perfectly with a Michael Scott *that's what she said* joke.

This show is the best, Marcus says, and catching him in a good mood, I remind him I need to take my mom to church in the morning.

I should probably leave after this episode.

I remind myself to never go on another date without my own car.

Marcus doesn't sing as much on the way back to my house, and he doesn't say he loves me again. He texts me the next day to tell me he's gotten back with his ex. I don't know if this is supposed to hurt me, but I feel relieved.

I still think about his animals sometimes.

I can't help myself.

Pennsboro, West Virginia, Calhoun's Tunnel, #7, 780 ft.

As I drive toward Pennsboro's half-deserted streets to search for Calhoun's Tunnel, I wonder about the bunker.

Like everything else in this county, you can't find anything about the bunker on the internet. Although I am kind of annoyed by this, I also love the lack of information. I enjoy the search for the unknown, and I appreciate a place in America actually exists where you can't find every single detail about it on the web.

From what I know about the bunker, it still exists somewhere near the old roller rink, where the women would come and go, skating with their high ponies swinging from their heads as they talked of Bruce Springsteen and The Cars and Bon Jovi, and I'm sure the people reading this from my home county have heard a hundred different other rumors about where the bunker actually is, but there's always a lot of talk and not quite as many answers.

The bunker? Near the gas station with the good slushies.

I do know where that place is—my mom loves the slushies.

The bunker? Twenty feet as the crow flies from Route 50, where that one exit used to be before they moved everything around, you know what I'm talking about.

No, sir, I have no clue.

The bunker? Just a little past where you turn off to go to Diane's house, where that oak tree is. It's underground there somewhere.

That's what my mom heard, but no one can seem to pin the location down on one of those West Virginia walls maps.

I'm also a Harrisvillian, which disqualifies me from knowing THE TRUTH (as Donald Trump might write) about the mysteries of Pennsboro, so as far as the bunker goes, I'm not sure what to do.

Much like these tunnels.

Calhoun's Tunnel, #7, doesn't pose as much of a navigational problem as some others have, but the entire trail welcomes me with five miles of a mud bath.

I've been losing weight, but on this trail, I'm nothing more than a slick pig writhing on a slaughtering table.

Although it's warm now, I'm still wearing my precious Keen boots I bought when I first moved to Boone in preparation for my inaugural mountain winter. Divorced and only responsible for myself, I was finally financially stable enough to buy something like winter boots. They cost more money than I should have spent, but they have lasted years and powered me through snowstorms and learning to walk again. As my former physical therapist Brad noted, boots offer more stability than sneakers, and he was damn right. I wouldn't want to walk through these tunnels with anything else on my feet but these snug snow boots.

Before I begin my hike through the tunnel, I glance at my phone and realize it's Dave's birthday. I once romanticized this date to an extreme. *If only I knew what happened to him, if only I knew where he was, if only if only if only.* I thought my life might improve if I could just find him and play out my lifelong fantasy of living with him and letting him take care of me, but it turned out that his damage far outweighed any love I thought I had for him.

I lost so much trust in myself after my imaginary relationship with Dave fell apart—because really, that's all Dave and I turned out to be.

Imaginary.

I imagined a person he might be, built him up in my head to an unhealthy extreme for two decades, and then allowed him back into my life at the most vulnerable time, without any idea of what he had been through or how he reacted, was reacting, and would react. I knew nothing about him, let my guard down after the whole pushing incident with CK, saw him as some kind of savior, and then let him in too quickly and easily without knowing anything about him at all.

I'm not convinced, though, that PTSD constituted the entire rage problem. I'm sure PTSD had something to do with it, but I'm just not willing to say that PTSD causes extreme bigotry and racism.

Because that is absolute horse shit, just like the horse shit mixed with all the mud here in Tunnel #7.

I dared to disturb that imaginary universe and unrequited love, therefore losing precious time.

However, I could have lost more. I could have spent even more time fantasizing about that bastard and even moved in with him. I could have been trapped with him in some house in some suburb of Virginia, wasting my numbered days being yelled at by a racist asshole.

I have never seen so much mud in a tunnel, and it's not even rainy or even misty today; it's gray, but that's typical for WV: green hills, gray sky. Welcome to the Mountain State, everyone. Hope you brought your trail mix and strong spirit because you're going to get hungry and depressed.

For the most part, these tunnels don't differ much. You

wander deep into the mouth, spend a few minutes meandering through the dark throat, and then you peregrinate out the other end like a time traveler. The fun, of course, is finding the tunnel, often popping up out of nowhere, on the trail, or better yet hiding shyly off to the side and slightly covered in grass, and wondering who tried the tunnel adventure before you. Who, in fact, didn't know this tunnel existed at all and was taken by surprise as they trekked here late one night, unaware of the strange comfort one can find in a passageway like this? Or who, like myself, came searching for answers they were unable to find within the passageways of their own brains and thoughts and sentiments?

I am too caught up in my musings to realize: I am stuck.

Not just a little stuck.

Like really fucking stuck in the Pennsboro mud on the opposite side of Calhoun's Tunnel.

I can't move my feet, and I'm sinking.

I panic. I can't die like this. I've been through way too much shit to choke in some quickmud in Pennsboro, West Virginia. That would be ridiculous. Has anyone ever died in quickmud? Is quickmud even a thing? As kids, we Xennials[5] always thought quicksand would be a huge problem in our lives; after all, cartoons made it seem that way. Sure, no one ever really had to deal with it as adults, not that I knew of, but maybe this was similar?

I'm going to have to get dirty.

I expect to get a bit fussed up, as we say here in West Virginia, when I hike in these tunnels, but today will be a *I need to do laundry before my parents see me* type of day, and I don't know how I'm going to pull that off.

I grab my phone from my pocket and toss it in the only dry patch of grass I see, which is a good ten feet away. By some miracle of lonesome trains past, my phone lands in that grass.

Naturally, I have zero service, so there's no calling for help. I'm not sure what I would do if someone did walk by. I half want some hiker to rip me out of this mud by the armpits and half want to die here of extreme embarrassment.

I plop my palms into some drier mud in front of me and finally gain some traction.

I will not die in the quickmud.

My mobility, better since I left North Carolina but not fantastic, fails me in this small-scale natural disaster. My left leg, typically strong enough to cover for my weak right leg, sinks knee-deep in this Appalachian trail mindfuck. I stop for a minute to take a few breaths; I wonder if anyone driving above on Route 50 can see me? If so, I hope they are laughing.

I cannot believe this shit.

With my hands, I endeavor to muscle my right leg out of the ground, but this feels like lifting a hundred pounds of dead weight from a well full of sand. My right arm, also weak since The Seizure That Ruined Everything, slides forward, and before I can use my left arm to assist, my face plops into the mud.

Well, this about says it all.

Horns echo above me.

I do not think they are beeping at me.

I imagine The Mothman. Why would I want some urban, granola hiker to rescue me? I would rather The Mothman swoop down with his glorious black wings, scoop me up from this mud pit, and let me fly around Appalachia with him, but I guess he's busy right now.

I am on my own, pinned, wriggling on this wall of dirt like a squished insect, going nowhere, just making some mud angels with my upper body, swimming in place in Pennsboro, West Virginia.

I rest for a moment, licking my tongue into the corners of

my muddy mouth. I am thirsty but don't have a water bottle with me on the trail; this is how hikers die. They get overconfident, forget their water, slip, fall, and no one ever sees them again.

Sure, they are on actual difficult, steep trails and not flat earth below an interstate, but details.

I have to rise. I have to get up.

I rest for another minute or so. Or is it an hour? In a second, there is time enough for an hour, it seems. Since *everything happened*, time has become as slippery as this quandary I've found myself in. I push myself up, downward-dog style, with every iota of energy I have, and my body makes a grotesque suctioning noise as I separate myself from the ground.

I've done it.

Sort of.

When I normally fall, this is how I get myself up, so my body is used to this. I can do it. My fingertips, ragged claws in this nasty mud, feel like the strongest part of my body right now. I know I need to extract my weak leg, the one that's only ankle deep, if I'm going to get out of this. I press my hands back into the mud and growl like a wild cat as I yank my leg as fast as I can from the spongy mess of ground.

I have one chance at this.

With my arms now elbow deep in the mud, I have to get this strong leg out, or I am finished.

The growling helps.

My left leg is free.

With my strong leg back in the wild, I'm able to pull my left arm out and rest again, still in downward dog position but with a couple free limbs. I've been half-bodied for a while now, so I feel normal, unless you consider I'm still half buried in the deep mud.

I don't think anyone walks on this trail, and if they do, it's not often.

But suddenly, I hear something.

I panic.

I don't know how I would possibly explain this. Would an able-bodied person end up in the mud like me? I think it's entirely possible. I'm not sure my disability had anything to do with my current precarious position. I start to wonder about my common sense. I don't have much, I admit, but as I glance around the trail, I notice I did take the best path. Except for the singular patch of grass I tossed my phone on, the other sections of trail are either swathed in dangerous branches I wouldn't be able to safely step over, inches deep of water, or also quick mud.

All those thoughts about wanting to have help were just insecurities. That isn't what I meant. I don't want help at all.

I am nearly free.

After my brief rest, I decide I should recline on my forearms to free my right leg. I pull as hard as I can with all the energy I can muster.

As it did with my left leg, this method works. I am perhaps stronger than I think.

There is one problem.

My right leg is free, but my boot is still stuck in the mud.

I consider trudging back to the car one-booted in my sock. I've never been happier to be separated from the ground. In all the falls I've had, and this was a necessary, planned collapse I've never been more thrilled to stand upright again.

But my boot.

It's been a good boot. I paid a lot of money for that boot, and when you're the type of person who was working three jobs[6] but still ate bruised bananas for every meal in grad school for a week straight because you couldn't afford to buy food for you and your pets and the pets came first, you don't leave something like that boot behind.

I try to dig the boot out with a stick.

No good.

Fuck it.

I scoop the mud out with my hands and finally have a boot again.

I don't even try to put the now-brown shoe back on my foot.

I have towels in my car.

I also have a banana, which I am still thankful for, despite those rough years of grad school.

When I arrive home, I am in luck. My mom is gone, probably somewhere with one of her many friends. Despite her stroke-related vision issues, that woman never misses a thing. She would absolutely die if she saw me walking in her new house more bog woman than mermaid, despite the mud being dried by now.

I roll up the bottom of my sweatpants and blaze past my dad, socks and boots in hand.

Hey, Suzanne, do you want some piz—

I strip my clothes off in the laundry room and toss them along with the boots in the washer. I can only hope for the best. The water turns from clear to black within seconds. The whir of the new washing machine sounds like faraway human voices as my boots drown in the chambers of three Tide Pods and domestic technology.

Calhoun's Tunnel still sings to me.

Harrisville, West Virginia

Neither Cathleen, Emily, nor I can find any of Attorney Tim's pictures online.

He's been texting me day and night about a *big trial* and

how important he is in *making stuff happen*. I get it. He's going through a divorce and needs attention; I'm happy to give it to him.

But.

Something is off.

Way off.

You can't exist today, especially as an attorney *involved in a big trial* in a state as small as West Virginia with zero online presence. I search news article after news article about trials in Charleston, and there are no Tims involved in any of them.

I need some help with this.

Cathleen guides me and Emily through a reverse Google image search, which seems easy when they do it on *Catfish*, but what Nev and Max/Kamie/whoever is co-hosting fail to mention is a reverse Google image search must be done on a desktop or laptop.

Not a phone.

Thank you, Cathleen, the only one in the cousin group who is Gen Z and certified in this knowledge.

Nothing comes up with the Tinder pics or photo of Burt the dog, but we have searched every law firm in Charleston (and the nearby areas), and there is no Tim or Timothy working for anyone. We can't even find a paralegal named Tim. To give him the benefit of the doubt, I suggest maybe it's a middle name.

We can check the WV state bar membership registry, Emily suggests in a group text with me and Cathleen. *Every state has one. It's public.*

Emily has a law degree and practiced for a minute before something better came up. She's brilliant.

I spend way too much time searching every single Tim, Timothy, and T. initial in the West Virginia State Bar Membership Portal that afternoon, and then I cross-reference them with

133

pics on attorney webpages. All of the Tim, Timothys, and T. initials are either way too old, established, married, or have some other anomaly making it impossible for the person I'm texting with to be named Tim.

I know.

I should have let it go.

But by now, you know me better than that.

There is nothing.

I spend the evening ignoring my phone and the tunnels to scour every single law firm's website in Charleston, which turns out to be quite a few. I search for a face match to a late-night selfie *Tim* sent me one night when he must have been drunk and forgetful that he sent me a selfie of someone different the previous week.

I'm still not sure where Tim works, so I start with the firms involved with *major trials* in the area to see if I can find a matching face for the late-night selfie.

Nope.

Nothing.

No results.

I will not give up. I will Nev Schulman this bastard until I find him.

That is unless he's not actually an attorney at all.

I have two law firms left on my list, and neither have had *big trials* in the paper.

I'm about to give up.

Then there he is.

Matthew Mitchell Mingoa.

I recognize the rosary he wears in his firm photo from the late-night selfie.

So Matthew, I text him. *How long were you planning on lying to me?* I send the text with a screenshot of his firm photo.

I screenshot the firm photo and selfie; I send the evidence to Emily and Cathleen.

TIMMATTHEW, Cathleen responds, and a nickname is born that he will never live down during our tumultuous hookupfriendshipsituation.

Well, well, well, congratulations. You figured it out, stalker, Timmatthew texts me.

Turns out I'm not your average online dater.

You'd be surprised how many girls figure it out.

Okay, I don't believe him for a second, and he's obviously **negging, *v.*: When men insult a woman with the purpose of lowering her self-esteem, hoping to make her more open to his later advances.**

He's angry I discovered his game so quickly.

I also know this isn't your real phone number.

Fine. It's a Google number.

He then gives me his actual number.

Although I should step away and step away faster than I have stepped away from anything before, I'm still semi-paralyzed, so I don't. That's a bad joke, but I don't know how else to explain why I put up with this prevarication for so long.

He looks exactly like an Italian-American Syed, Cathleen texts.

Syed is her ex-boyfriend who is so terrible her friends call him Syed-19.

He does, Emily adds.

Why did you lie like that? I ask Timmatthew.

I need to know.

Eh, it's because I had a bad experience with a girl on Tinder not so long ago. She was crazy! I turned her down, and she stalked everything—sent me hundreds of texts, called me nonstop, called my work number, and even used my work email.

135

I couldn't get away from her. So, it just seemed easier to start off very vague.

But it wasn't vague. It was a straight-up lie.

I guess so.

Well, I don't really know what to do from here.

I'd like to keep talking to you.

I guess I have nothing better to do because although I'd like to say I cut him completely off, I did not. I kept talking to him. I met up with him. I imagined we would date, and he would represent me in some *big trial* where we would figure out who was responsible for my brain cancer, and we would win lots of money and live together happily ever after in some reverse Erin Brockovich fantasy.

That's not what happened, of course.

What happened was we hooked up a few times, and each time, I thought it was going to lead to something more than what it ever did.

What happened was he promised to make me a table (he does woodworking in his spare time) with The Owl Picture in the center. The Owl Picture is a sentimental, kitschy piece of art my grandmother featured in my aunt's bedroom, where Emily and I hung out when we went to visit. If Emily went and I wasn't visiting that weekend or vice versa, we left letters for one another behind The Owl Picture. When our grandmother died, Emily rescued The Owl Picture from her crumbling house, and we started mailing the actual picture back-and-forth. Then we realized it was popular in thrift stores and found our own replicas.

Somehow, we both ended up with two.

I mailed Timmatthew an Owl Picture from Etsy, and he promised to make me a table from it, and you guessed it—never saw that table.

What happened was I still occasionally text him for whatever reason, though I guess we became friends of some sort.

What happened was I didn't really have anyone else with that kind of time.

Salem, WV, kinda, Brandy Gap Tunnel, #2, 1086 ft.

I can't figure out how to find this tunnel at all.

One of the furthest ones from my parents' house (it still doesn't feel like my house at all, not really), the directions I have pieced together from various sources on the internet lead me to the side of Route 50.

Okay, sure. I pull my trusty tiny Scion into the grass and hope no state troopers will find an eggplant-colored miniature car pulled off into the grass beside a major highway suspicious. If they do, my parents will for sure hear about it before I get home.

The amalgam of GPS directions I have on scraps of paper have led me into the woods. I wander around like a spirit for a few minutes. The tunnel could be here, after all, but I soon realize I am not in the correct place. I retreat back to the tiny Scion for a moment, the only place lately I have truly felt at home, and then I decide to drive up the grass a bit and try a different spot in the woods. After piecing together my puzzle of paper scraps, it seems I'm just a few tenths of a mile from where I need to be.

It's 1539 all over again, and I am a female Hernando de Soto, modernized in my Old Navy sweatpants and Keen boots, discovering the Appalachian Mountains for the first time.

Okay, fine, I am nothing like that, but I need some adventure in my life, so I pretend I am seeking something no one else has found before, and if I have to tromp through some woods on the side of the so-called Loneliest Road in America (which is actually pretty busy in the daylight hours) to do it, so be it.

Maybe no one will notice my shiny purple car?

I pull up a bit, careful I don't get stuck in any ditches. I can't imagine the embarrassment of calling a tow truck for this and what my dad might say about it. He would never have to know, but this news always gets around Harrisville.

Fast.

I wander around the woods for a moment. I should have had a snack, but I regret nothing. Who wouldn't want to stomp around the woods in the middle of a warm afternoon and then happen upon an abandoned tunnel? I'd be lying if I said I didn't hope one day I might step into one of those tunnels and never come out; I wouldn't even necessarily care where I ended up or why—just anywhere but the side of Route 50.

Maybe I would end up on the side of a mountain, a sunny place with no brain cancer or consistently gray skies. I would live in a log cabin that smelled like bacon and have no Wi-Fi or need for it. I would just walk and take care of cats all day long, and what a life that would be. The love of my life would never talk to me but cook me bacon and live a life all his own.

Maybe I would end up in a different time period, Victorian London perhaps, where I would work for a newspaper with Emily. We would write human interest stories all day and care to do nothing else. Both of us would die within days of one another in our 60s, therefore eliminating the need for either of us to be sad.

Maybe I would end up in a house I see in my dreams all the time, a red house with windows all the way around the building. It's an ominous house, but I feel comfortable here. I've been here many times before. There is no furniture, not now anyway. A dark basement. I will always come back here.

Okay, before I know it, I'm a little lost elf in the woods, and

I see no tunnel. Sure, most tunnels are on the Rail Trail, but I have very little information about this one, and I forgot to write down whether it had been bypassed. I realize with disappointment I might have fucked up the whole thing; the tunnel might have been daylighted, meaning the roof has been removed, and it's...not actually a tunnel anymore.

I did remember to begin my mile tracker, which works whether I have cell service or not, and I hardly ever do. I have zigzagged about a mile from the highway, and I worry my car won't be there when I get back. Honestly, a state trooper could pick that thing up and throw it to the nearest tow service if they wanted to, and though this would make my life way more exciting, it would truly screw me over because there is no way my parents would be able to pick me up, and Ubers and Lyfts do not exist here.

As I trudge through the leaves, mucky and wet from the West Virginia weather, I wish to see a squirrel or deer or something, but I am alone. I don't see any tunnel or path leading to a tunnel. I wonder if I have made a grave mistake, and this tunnel is gone for good.

No, I tell myself.

I may have brain damage, but I wouldn't have made a mistake like that.

I wander around for a few more minutes before I think I've lost my car. The state troopers have found it and impounded it. I'm going to have to call Mr. Samples and let him rag on me for a minute before agreeing to send someone to pick me up. Probably our family friend Michelle, who will laugh at me about the whole thing.

But as it happens, I'm just turned around, and the tiny Scion is right where I left it.

I wait until there are zero cars on the highway and pull onto the road. For a giant's roller skate, the acceleration is better than one might expect. I'm waiting to be pulled over, but somehow, I survive the blue and red lights of any bored cop.

I take myself to the Clarksburg Starbucks and sit in the car, eating fancy cheese and drinking a refresher.

It would be an embarrassment to drive home at this point.

Huntington, West Virginia

To get out of Harrisville, I visit my Aunt Tammy (Emily's mom) and her sister Tiffany near Huntington, where I lived during college and grad school. They reside outside of the city, next to a miniature goat farm. When I pull up to their house, the baby goats, just born last month, run to me gleefully, bleating and welcoming me to the farm.

It's the warmest hello I've ever experienced.

When we visit the goats later, a little one named George allows me to feed him animal crackers, pick him up, and hold him for over four minutes, which seems like a record for a baby goat.

Tammy moved in with Tiffany after my Uncle Roger died and Tiffany's husband, Randy, suffered debilitating, life-altering injuries in a work accident. Tiffany tried caring for him at home and created a handicapped-accessible basement for him, but eventually, it all became too much. His caregivers were stealing his medication and Tiffany's things. When she had to fire the caregivers, Tiffany couldn't work and pay the bills. Eventually, Randy went to live at a long-term care center, and Tiffany visits him at least once a day.

I know people say that shit all the time, but she is there at least once a day, but most of the time, more.

That woman has never wavered.

When I get inside, Aunt Tammy tells me what I need to know.

And there is *a lot* to know.

Tam & Tiff, living as two single women, do not take *being alone* lightly. Aunt Tammy tells me their *favorite things to watch on TV are Little House on the Prairie and Criminal Minds*, and every bit of this house shows it. Both employed by Hobby Lobby, the seasonal pillows and decorations are in full rotation. Although I'm there after July 4th and there's no real holiday to celebrate, they have the bottom floor, the handicapped-accessible spot, decked out in summer vibes. I know for sure they did not do this for me—they would have decorated down here regardless.

Tam Tam—as she is affectionally known—gives me the rundown when I arrive.

There are cameras everywhere.

Originally, Tiff had her son install the cameras to dissuade Randy's nurses from stealing, but once Randy was transferred to the caregiving facility, everyone agreed it was beneficial to leave them up. The other day, Tiff found car tracks in the yard, so the outside cameras are especially beneficial to make sure no one—and I mean NO ONE—messes with the sisters. Their father was a cop, so yes, they have some of his old guns, and Tiffany dang sure knows how to use them, but they would prefer not to. If I happen to have *a special someone*, he is welcome to come over (if I wouldn't mind giving Tam Tam some info about him, like his social security number, parents' names, his place of employment, and past three landlord references), but no friends.

Luckily for them, I do not have *a special someone*, and I have plans to meet up with friends, but only within the limits of Huntington proper. I wouldn't dare invite guests to a house where I'm already a guest, and I write that without a salt of sarcasm.

Tam Tam has prepared a giant bowl of sugar free banana

pudding for me and somehow found sugar free Ale-8s from where she used to live in Kentucky.

I nearly weep.

It's been such a long time since someone has done something so nice for me.

I have zero cell phone service here and have to drive to the gas station down the road to text anyone; this is the perfect vacation.

I may be in Tam Tam & Tiff's Foucauldian Appalachian Panopticon, but I will be well fed and watered.

If I need anything while they are at work, I'm welcome to use the house phone and rely on the dogs for company.

Wendy: an ornery Shiatzu who loves sitting in my lap, especially when I have snacks.

Moses: a gentle giant Great Pyrenees who wakes me up when my blood sugar plummets in the middle of the night.

Pebbles: a miniature something-or-other whose tongue does not stay in her mouth. I can't remember her name and keep calling her Penny. Petunia. Pistachio. She doesn't answer to any of them.

They are my new best friends.

I wonder if my Tinder roster will miss me this weekend, but I honestly don't care. I need a break. It's a lot to keep up with, and they've all been ***breadcrumbing, v.*: the act of leading someone on with no real intention of meeting up or dating them, like dropping breadcrumbs,** me lately. I wish I had never become familiar with the term, but sadly, it became my present reality while hunkering down in Harrisville for the past six months.

Anything is better than Dave, though.

Anything is better than those early morning screaming phone calls.

Loneliness.

Anything.

Before Tam Tam absconds to Hobby Lobby, she wants to *warn me about one thing.*

We have a violent neighbor, she says.

The violent neighbor owns a tattoo parlor on the main drag, and the violent neighbor has violent dogs.

Sometimes Tam Tam & Tiff fire warning shots with their Pop's old gun.

He won't bother you, though, she assures me as she adjusts her Hobby Lobby apron.

I'm starting to wonder.

I have the Wi-Fi password and consider if I even want to use it.

I sit in Grey Gardens 2.0 and wonder what to do next.

* * *

After telling my life story to some baby goats through the fence, I go to the gas station and text Travis. We had plans to meet up tonight and despite my lack of cell service, I know unlike my Tinder roster, Travis will not let me down.

Target parking lot at 5? I text.

Sounds like a plan.

We meet up, and nothing has changed.

Well, everything has changed, but our friendship hasn't.

I hop in his car (as much as I can hop in my current state), and he gives me a driving tour of where he grew up. I feel like I'm on the set of *The Wonder Years.*

That's where I lived, he says as he points to any house in any nondescript neighborhood, but this one happens to be special because it's his. *And over there is where Josh grew up.*

Josh.

The One Who Got Away.

I can't remember the last time I spoke to Josh, but he did contact me When Everything Happened, which I thought was nice. Despite me being mad at him for a while when I left for grad school over a decade ago—I seriously thought we could maintain a long-distance relationship with him in West Virginia and me in Alabama—I didn't have any negative feelings toward him and hadn't for a long time.

I'd always hoped he was happy and occasionally liked his Instagram stories.

I'm sure Dave would have loved that.

We used to jump from the top of that hill there and slide to the bottom, Travis tells me.

I can picture this frame-by-frame, like I'm watching old home movies. My communication with Travis always has this nostalgic effect on me.

We continue the drive to Travis and Josh's old middle and high schools, where one of my baton-twirling friends, Jamie, briefly dated Travis.

And that is where Jamie and I shared all of our deepest secrets! Travis jokes. He parks at the football field. *Our football captain was super talented but got into drugs, bad. He killed himself on the field, I think. Actually, I might have made that whole story up.*

We both laugh. Our humor is a bit dark sometimes.

We drive and drive and drive.

We go past his little brother's old log cabin in the woods.

We go past the *motherfucking Bojangles* that somehow failed. (What's wrong with you, Huntington?)

We go past the city limits.

Travis is one of the only people I feel safe around. I can be myself. I can talk. I can be quiet. I can be bitchy. I can be whatever I want.

I'm sure he feels the same with me.

Somehow, we end up in South Charleston.

You should text Timmatthew, Travis jokes. *I bet he's in the garage with a saw, making you a table.*

We can't hold it in; we are in hysterics.

When Travis speaks, I always picture the story happening in front of me. It's a bond created by two writers.

I do text Timmatthew, but as more of a joke than anything else.

I'm in South Charleston with Travis!

Is that the friend or the other guy you're talking to?

Sounds like someone might be jealous.

I leave the text alone for a moment.

I've never driven through South Charleston before.

It's as gray as old donkey fur but wetter and more miserable.

I let my mind wander a bit. What if Timmatthew was free and wanted to meet up with me and Travis? That might be fun. We could have a couple drinks in South Charleston.[7] Travis could give me his (dis)approval before driving us back to the Target parking lot.

I know this will never happen, but Timmatthew is the best romantic hope I have at the moment. I just want *something* so badly.

I don't want to die alone.

Everyone knows that.

Timmatthew shows the most interest, and sure, he did ghost me for an entire weekend (well, he said *I got buried,* which was an interesting choice of words considering my situation), and sure, he was definitely avoidant and gave absolutely zero indication of wanting a serious relationship with me, but he did know what I was looking for and chose to proceed, so that had to mean something, right?

Travis isn't so sure.

I just don't want you to get hurt, and I... I've been around enough guys like him to see where this is headed.

You think it's headed nowhere.

I just don't think it's going where you want it to go.

I know Travis is right; he's usually right. I also know what you might be thinking—is Travis single? Why don't you two just burn that friendship to the ground for good and actually give it a shot?

No.

Well, we do joke about that, but it's not going to happen.

Travis knows what's going to happen next.

So...how's Josh?

I instantly feel guilty for asking, but I need to know.

Travis understands.

He's okay. He and that girl he was seeing broke up.

I didn't have to say anything.

Do you think it would be okay if I sent him a text?

Oh yeah, I think he'd like hearing from you.

I must admit, this car ride has me feeling sentimental, and I don't care a whole lot about my Tinder roster now, even Timmatthew there at the top. Knowing Josh is single gives me a different kind of hope, and my heart is revived. Imagining Josh and Travis jumping down that hill, *Wonder Years* style, makes me feel very Winne Cooper, albeit less whiny, or at least I would like to think so.

I don't know if Josh will be able to meet up, and I don't want anything physical from him. It would just be nice to have a reminder that at one time, I had chemistry with someone. Before I became a diseased, defunct, broken human, I actually clicked with someone very organically, without all the online messiness, and we liked each other and had a brief romantic fling before I drove to Alabama with nothing in my car but some clothes and a cat.

Josh and I never slept together—a debate we once had a couple years after I left that he had to consult his journals about because he swore we did—but this somehow made the experience more meaningful to me.

Travis introduced us briefly by happenstance at Starbucks. I was with my mom and Nana, who had come to help me after a mono diagnosis kicked my ass during my last fall semester of grad school. I was feeling better, so we went out to eat. Somehow, my blood sugar dropped, so we stopped to get a drink, and Travis and Josh were there. The introduction was brief but meaningful.

I later accompanied Travis to an art show Josh was having in a nearby Kentucky town, and the three of us spent the evening goofing off, discussing photography, and gazing at the stars at a nearby park. We discussed John Titor, the time traveler from the year 2036, who posted on obscure message boards we somehow all knew about. We bit the ears off chocolate bunnies while Josh documented the night in black and white.

The evening changed me.

Josh and I embarked on a flirtatious few months that I, naturally, took as more than it was supposed to be, which was a theme that would continue for the remainder of my adulthood.

It was definitely a *situationship, n.*: **A type of relationship where one person wants a commitment, and the other person simply wants sex or a hookup. The person pursuing the relationship will likely try different unsuccessful approaches, such as suggesting actual dates, playing house, or meeting each other's friends, while the other**

person is likely to only text or call at night and suggest hooking up.

I only blamed Josh for about two weeks before I decided I needed to take some responsibility for myself and my own actions.

Although I was in my mid-20s, I couldn't distinguish casual romantic relationships from falling in love, and two months before I left, I found myself wishing my situationship with Josh could be an actual relationship.[8] The opposite of me, Josh is magnetic in a way I've only ever experienced with my sister. I would go out to meet Josh at the V Club in Huntington, and he would be surrounded by people at all times, his long blonde hair in a ponytail and rakish good looks offset by his insistence on dressing exactly like Eddie Vedder.

His popularity didn't bother or dissuade me, though. After growing up with Sarah, I was quite accustomed to playing the prop friend. I liked the role, actually. If someone wanted to talk to me, great, but if they didn't, I was happy to soak in the noise and conversation around me like a strawberry drowning in vodka, the drink settling in my hand.

After having fun at the bar one night, I expected to go home alone, but Josh offered to drive me back. That night, I locked myself out—a rather frequent occurrence if I am being honest. I always attributed this to being a scatter-brained writer, but knowing what I know now, I understand I likely already had a brain tumor causing me major memory issues. I instructed Josh to follow me up the fire escape so I could open up the unlocked kitchen window and crawl in. We hooked up on my floor mattress, only there because I was moving soon and had sold all my furniture, and I would see this as one of the most romantic moments of my life.

How could I not?

And then a few days later, Josh began ignoring my

Myspace messages and texts. When I saw him at the V Club, he said *I really wish you weren't leaving*, and I lost my mind. I yelled at Josh outside of the bar and drove around a few hours, crying and wondering if Travis had any drugs he could give me.

I didn't think I would make it to Auburn at this rate.

Later the same night, I found an article about Conor Oberst from the band Bright Eyes in a music magazine I bought at the local bookstore and wrote Josh some really weird note on the pages. I tore them out, put them on his car, and didn't see him again for a few more years.

Thanks for the note on my car, he texted a few days later, but I knew it was over.

My good friend Betsy, who had hung out with both of us at the bar, saw him at The V Club months after I left and said, *How's Suzanne?* and he responded, *Which one?*

Betsy, who has always been honest with me, told me the whole thing, and because my only friend at Auburn so far was Michael Scott from *The Office*, what Betsy told me was devastating.

I was glad she told me, though.

I needed to hear it.

* * *

I decide to spend a couple nights in a downtown Huntington hotel.

I want to see a couple of friends, safely of course.

Although I had tons of fun at Grey Gardens 2.0, it's not really a conducive space to meeting up with anyone.

I want to see Betsy, the same friend who gave me intel about Josh, and her ex-husband Jesse. I'm friends with Betsy because of Jesse, but when they divorced, I remained friends with both.

I met Jesse my freshman year at Marshall University. I was scared of him because he wore a black trench coat and wrote stories about people with Body Integrity Identity Disorder, or people who desire to become amputees. I was fresh out of Christian small-town America, and this terrified me. America was also only a couple years post-Columbine, and back then, school shootings were still an anomaly. Trench coats + Boys Who Wrote Creepy Short Stories= Potential School Shooters.

I couldn't take any chances.

Jesse was actually the opposite of this, though, and once I stopped judging everyone I met, we became good friends. When he told me he had a girlfriend I would love, I imagined a gothic gal obsessed with tumblr and Japanese culture (not that there's anything wrong with this), but Betsy was a trendy, curly-haired showstopper who never failed to call me out on my bullshit, buy me trendy makeup for Christmas, and dish on the latest celebrity gossip with me.

Jesse was right.

I loved her.

She was and is the coolest.

And maybe, just maybe during this hotel stay, I would see Josh.

I don't know what I'm expecting to happen.

Probably nothing.

I also have an MRI in Charleston, WV, in two days.

My doctor says it's fine, that because of Covid, I can do my MRI in Charleston, then have an awkward telehealth appointment about my fantastic results. I won't have to stay in a gross Winston-Salem hotel that smells of rotting bus seats. I'll miss the Bojangles, but in the end, it will be less time and money and therefore, worth it.

My parents know about the MRI but have said nothing.

I do a quick grand Huntington tour of hanging out with

both Betsy and her new husband and Jesse and his new wife, all of which is lovely. I get a bit too drunk by the time I'm at Jesse's and end up hugging him and crying because *I never thought I would see him again since I thought I was going to die three years ago,* and it's dramatic but goddammit, it's all true. I really do miss my friends in Huntington and wish I would have stayed there sometimes, but I really wanted that Ph.D., though all the good it's done me is get me in a lot of debt.

I'm finally buzzed enough to text Josh.

Hey! Travis gave me your number. I probably had it somewhere. Actually, I had it memorized, but I wasn't sure it was still yours. Anyway. I'm in town. I'm not sure what your situation is. I'd love to hang out. No worries if you can't.

I'm not sure if that's actually what I texted, but it was something of the sort.

And for once, I truly mean what I say. I'm tired enough to go to bed if he's busy. Although I haven't spoken to Josh in years, I imagine he's still the same popular, beloved, out-on-the-town guy I knew a decade ago.

He texts back like he's been waiting for me.

Yeah, I'm down. What do you want to do? Where are you?

I'm confused.

I don't remember a time when a love interest, flirtatious or serious, actually responded so straightforwardly, Josh included.

And there is no situation.

I text him I'm staying at the Marriott, and we can meet up soon to get a drink or something. I'm very nonspecific. This is what happens after a month of online dating ruins your soul; you start being as indifferent with your plans as Elon Musk is with hundred-dollar bills.

Okay, I think. I am moving forward so far. I know better, though. I cannot get too excited here. I don't know anything about Josh these days. I'm looking for something real, something serious. If he's anything like he was when I knew him before, it's doubtful he is. And, if I'm putting this together correctly, his last relationship didn't end that long ago, so it wouldn't be right to pressure him into anything or even bring up the possibility.

But still.

I think of that night in his art studio.

Do you think this picture is too personal or would you try to sell it? he asked me, minutes after we met. I was going to my grandmother's funeral the next day and almost didn't accompany Travis, but in the end thought, *why the hell not?* My Grandma Samples was a practical person, and it would not have been practical to sit in my apartment alone. *I'd definitely try to sell it,* I told him. *Sure, it's personal, but it's beautiful. You're really talented.* The black and white photograph was of an ex and clearly of her either waking up in the morning or of him on top of her while fucking. I felt like someone actually valued my opinion on something I knew nothing about, which made me feel way more important than I should have. *Yeah, I'll try to sell it,* he said. *Definitely display it.*

I think of nights at the V Club, Josh catching my eye across the bar and smiling while entertaining a conversation with eight other people I'd never seen before. *Have you ever met ALPHABET SOUP?* he would ask me, the names too jumbled for me to hear. I didn't know any of them; well, I actually would know some of them, but usually I would pretend I didn't to avoid the awkwardness of admitting how I did know them, which was because we had all hooked up with the same people at some point or another.

Josh was just so innocent in his interactions.

All of them.

I think of making out with him on the mattress in my old apartment, always imagining I'd never see him again.

We probably shouldn't sleep together, both of us agreed. *It will just make things harder*, and then it was over faster than the Bright Eyes song on my Myspace profile, something I would cringe at now.

After dillydallying at Starbucks for a good hour or so, I walk into the Marriott and give a quick hi to the receptionist, who looks bored enough to play Solitaire on her work computer. I hope to get some rest in my room and do myself up a bit before meeting Josh.

I sigh as I step onto the elevator. I'm a bit tired. A guy wearing cowboy boots runs on at the last second, and he seems to be in the mood for conversation.

I am not.

So, you have any plans tonight? the stranger asks. *Going out anywhere?*

I roll my eyes. I can't help it. I'm annoyed.

He's attractive enough with his chiseled jaw, but I'm tapped out. I need to recharge before talking to anyone else. Even the crowd at Starbucks, whom I didn't interact with, and the bored receptionist wore me down. I grimace as I realize he didn't ask me to press any other elevator button.

He's on my floor.

I sigh again, heavier this time. I need him to really notice I'm not in the mood. If I was going out, which I am, with Josh, it's not going to be with him.

Definitely staying in tonight, I say, careful to avoid eye contact. *My friend is coming over.*

The stranger grabs my arm. Holy shit. I've heard of stuff like this happening, but in the Huntington Marriott? Really? I am about ready to reach for the emergency button in the elevator and give the bored Marriott employee something to enliven her evening.

Suzanne, it's me.

Oh my god. Josh. You—oh my god, you look so different.

We awkwardly get off on the 11th floor. The good thing about knowing someone for this long is that this type of discomfort will dissipate into something different in a matter of moments. It won't last long.

I can only hope.

I am incredibly embarrassed.

Probably my most embarrassing moment ever.

Like, ever.

A few hours ago, I was fantasizing about living out my forever with this guy, and then I didn't even recognize him face-to-face in the elevator. This is not how I imagined meeting Josh again. I suppose I wanted him to run up to me in the hotel lobby after I had rested an hour or so and prepared myself, put on some makeup for godssake, and fixed my hair a bit. After all these years, a cancer diagnosis, a kind-of-remission, toxic relationships, a pandemic, and moving home with my parents, I wanted a moment.

Well, I guess in a way I got one.

I am so sorry. Oh my god.

He is cracking up.

I can't look at him.

To be fair, I did find you attractive in the elevator. I was just thinking, this dude needs to realize, I'm meeting up with my friend Josh, and I have no interest in him!

Oh, so you did find me attractive?

I did, but I was set on hanging out with...you tonight. I wasn't about to give my number to some handsome stranger.

I'm finally able to look at him again.

I don't feel like I aged well, Josh says, but I disagree. He does look different, but in the best way. He doesn't dress like Eddie Vedder anymore. Gone are the spandex leggings under jeans shorts— Josh has replaced them with actual jeans and, of course, the cowboy boots. He has glasses now and didn't before. He still has the long hair, but it's a bit darker.

Still blonde but darker.

The cowboy boots make him a lot taller.

I think you look more distinguished.

Thanks. That makes me feel good.

I'm still fucking embarrassed, I say, and we both laugh.

The chemistry is still there.

We sit in my hotel room and fall into an easy conversation. Nothing serious, nothing strange. It's like we didn't lose touch for seven years.

So, you wanna get out of here? he asks.

I don't know. I said that guy in the elevator I was staying in because my friend was coming over.

We laugh.

Of course, I say, and we walk out into the city night. This feels familiar, like the evening after the art show. I feel like we have traveled back into time aboard John Titor's spaceship, but this is all for selfish purposes, and neither of us care. It's impractical, and we know it, like people who have dashed through galaxies all for the sake of love and love alone.

He grabs my hand, and I let him.

I feel a freedom I haven't felt since I was in my early 20s.

The night is ours.

* * *

After a few cocktails, Josh walks me back to the hotel room. He holds my hand like a father holds a kid's hand, and I think nothing of it. I'm having trouble walking, so I feel like he's just helping me out.

I only cried once throughout our drinks.

A record for me.

I enjoy every moment with Josh and don't think about the next one. As a responsible, anxious planner with cancer, this is a new experience for me. I am not accustomed to this luxury. With him, I don't think about what could be or what might happen next.

I simply enjoy the moment and my drink and his conversation.

He asks *what happened*, but only in a way Josh could. He thinks differently than anyone else I know, and this is a good thing. As an artist, his strokes are broad and colorful. He doesn't feel sorry for me or ask what comes next; he just listens and drinks alongside me, which is exactly what I need right now.

We sit in the hotel room, the elevator stranger and I, and I assume he will leave at any moment. I am okay with this, in a way I would only be with Josh and not with anyone else. A Tinder date would leave me feeling nervous and wondering *what would happen next*, but with him, I would be fine if he gave me a hug and said, *see you next time.*

So, do you want to cuddle up?

I ask him to repeat himself because I assume he's going to leave and make this another *what if* moment I can fantasize about the final years of my life. It's nice like this, I tell myself, these romantic *what ifs* that never materialize. As I'm dying in a hospital somewhere, I'll think about this sweet moment with Josh and remember all the *almosts* and *maybes* and how I complained about Father John Misty playing at the bar because even though he's someone *I should be into, I just can't stand him* and Josh said, *That's an odd thing to say*, but he smiled a little, and I didn't feel weird for telling him any of it.

And I'll remember how just like at the V Club years ago, Josh knew everyone at the nameless bar across the street from the hotel, across from the Starbucks where we met ten years ago, and this turns me on, but I say nothing. I just sit and watch him stir his drink, and only Josh could sip such a girly cocktail and still look masculine somehow, just like he can wear the cowboy boots and somehow not look redneck or anything like a cowboy.

Do you want to get in bed with me?

In a hotel beside the Starbucks where we first met, we open our cassette in complete darkness and begin to develop the old films we have packed away for so long, slowly, and carefully so we don't destroy any images.

Here we were.

Here we are.

Better than before.

We climb into bed, and he holds me.

Nothing has changed.

Everything has changed.

It's late, and we are both tipsy, but I don't care. I remember this feeling of being loved, cared for. Something tells me it won't last, but in this moment, it's worth it, every bright color from 3rd avenue in Huntington fading to black-and-white, every moment blossoming on the film.

Charleston Area Medical Center, Charleston, West Virginia

I show up for my MRI in plenty of time, and after my tour of the goat farm and Huntington's 3rd Avenue, I almost forget my real reason for being here. As a meemaw and peepaw-type couple discuss wanting a Tudor's biscuit after Peepaw's procedure this morning, I remember what it's like to live in West Virginia. *I wanna Mary B*, Peepaw says, and honestly, that would be my choice, too.

I'm fucking hungry.

I am called back for the MRI, but being *called back* means walking five feet to a curtained-off area. The woman who tries to insert the IV for my MRI, a definite lesbian with a buzzed haircut, left-arm tattoo sleeve, and she/her on her nametag, brightens my day when she touches my arm and says, *I can tell we are going to be friends*. I start doubting my sexuality hard when this happens, but then I remind myself I don't have to decide.

I can date whomever I want, whenever I want, blah blah blah. It just so happens at this point, West Virginia is a wasteland of single lesbians, and ~~going either way~~ going *all the ways* and seeing *people for people and not sex organs* allow me to meet and connect with people as they are and not what they're like in bed.

I'm far more interested in the former.

But anyway, no one can get my IV in, same old story, and the woman tells me *I thought we were gonna be friends, Suzanne,* and smiles at me with eyes the color of the Kanawha[9] River (though perhaps this is an unfair comparison because she has quite nice eyes and that river is polluted and awful). Eventually, someone else gets in the IV, and I look for the woman on Tinder that afternoon but never find her.

I also never got my Tudor's biscuit, but I hope Peepaw got his Mary B.

Charleston, West Virginia

I didn't plan this, but I'm meeting up with Timmatthew while I'm in Charleston, and I'm definitely going to sleep with him.

Although I haven't met Timmatthew yet, and yes, he did catfish me and it was a shitty thing to do and I kinda hate him for it, he's good conversation. He did ghost me that one weekend, but he has twin toddler daughters and he's an attorney in Charleston, so it seemed acceptable, expected even, and now he texts back with regularity and efficiency.

I have this weird attraction to him I can't explain.

Once I busted him on the Google phone number and he gave me his actual phone number, we kept texting on both. He pretended to be a werewolf and I was a lady in love with very furry men, and then I would text his actual phone number and tell Timmatthew about this bizarre guy who was pretending to be a werewolf and wouldn't leave me alone.

It was weird.

It was fun.

It was everything cancer wasn't.

I'd never been in this position before. More than one guy (three if you counted the werewolf) had an interest in me, but none actually had taken the next step to be in a defined relationship. I had made clear to everyone, at least in general terms, that I was concerned with relationships and not hookups. I didn't want to have someone in bed with me one night and like a ghost in a tunnel, gone the next.

Josh was a surprise, so he gets a pass.

Did I have to try out different people in bed to get to the next step? It's not something I wanted to do, but I felt as if I had been the one making all the definite moves, and I was starting to get really sick of it.

I wait for Timmatthew in the hotel bar at the Charleston Town Center Marriott and have this feeling I'm going to get ghosted. I order a gin and tonic, a drink we both spoke of liking. The bartender gives me a sad glance, like he realizes I'm about to get ghosted, too. The drink arrives in a foggy glass, and I think of the tunnels.

The MRI is over; I'll just celebrate on my own.

How much time have I spent in hotels since my diagnosis?

Too much, but I don't mind. Every hotel feels like home. The Tallest Man on Earth's "Hotel Bar" plays in my mind. Halfway through my drink, I see whom I believe to be Timmatthew amble past the large hotel bar picture windows. (It's hard to tell with someone who has catfished you. Did they really ever send an accurate picture? Did they?) But it is him, and I give him an easy Suzanne smile that everyone gets, and he orders a bottled beer.

The bartender looks relieved he doesn't have to console another patron for being stood up. How many people has he had to listen to? *I don't know what happened...she said she would meet me here and then she just never...I'll have another beer.* Naturally, the confessions only come after the first three drinks, after they've been waiting at least thirty minutes.

Timmatthew is handsome enough, but I still can't quite figure out why I've pinned so many romantic hopes on him. Sure, we like the same kind of music. Sure, he has a good sense of humor. Sure, he's intelligent. But this isn't exactly like me to pursue someone who lied to me for a couple of weeks about who he was, and he's not even my physical type. He's lanky with green eyes, dark hair, and definitely got that cool/nerdy vibe about him, but I left that type behind in grad school. This feels like a regression, but I like him and can't figure out why.

I don't know why I'm thinking so much about this.

I like him because he pays attention to me and then he backs off.

It's the classic cat-and-mouse game.

He openly hates cats but is one.

How could I like someone who doesn't love cats?

I ask Timmatthew why he didn't order a gin-and-tonic. Since we had this conversation about how we both love the drink (plus, the villains in his favorite movie adore the cocktail), and he looks at me like I'm eight shots deep and doing karaoke with the Amazing Delores[10] in a dive bar downtown.

I've always hated those, he says, looking me right in the eye.

I don't have the greatest memory because of *the brain issues* and I'm prone to fantasy, so maybe, just perhaps, I created all this about both of us loving gin-and-tonics. There is a far greater chance, however, he said this to me in passing through text one night and thought I wouldn't remember it.

For someone with a fourth of my frontal lobe missing, I still have a fantastic memory.

I let it go.

I just want to feel something tonight.

Anything.

Timmatthew is on his phone; obviously not a fan of this behavior, I ask what's so important. The only acceptable answer I can think of would be something to do with his daughters.

Oh, I'm checking out my horses. I haven't told you about this yet, but I'm part owner of a racehorse. I like to bet on the ponies. I won a grand the other day!

It's hard to ignore his excitement. I'm not a fan of the way racehorses are treated, but like everything else men have done lately, I let it slide in the name of *giving him a chance.* His passion for something, anything, turns me on, and I suddenly get in my head we will take this date up to my hotel room and at least make out a little.

Have some fun.

We don't have to, you know, fuck or fall in love, but anything in between would be nice. After my ultra-romantic night in Huntington with Josh, I haven't heard from him at all. He didn't wish me luck with the MRI, driving home, nothing. Not that he owed me anything, but I kind of felt like he would at least wish me well. We didn't end my trip with any declarations of love, but at the end of the day, Josh and I have always been friends, and I would wish my friend a good MRI.

I suddenly feel badly for thinking Timmatthew was on his phone texting other women or worse yet, swiping on the dating apps. He was simply excited about a passion, and if it was happening during our date, who was I to stop him? I flag down the bartender for another gin and tonic and give him the glare of *see? He showed up, and I guarantee he will end up in my room tonight.*

He brings me another, and I should probably slow down.

Boozanne Shambles is back in town.

Timmatthew's words make me spin round-and-round.

I've always been horrible at poetry.

Timmathew is a bit more awkward than I expected, louder and as nasally as my college boyfriend, but we make interesting conversation, or try to, at least. He's mentioned to me yet again how the last girl *he was talking to was crazy and stalked him, bombing his work email and phone. That's why he had to give me a Google number and catfish me.* I mean, all women are crazy, right? Haven't we all heard that?

I don't know why I still like him. Women have heard all these excuses before, but there's something deeply broken inside of me since CK pushed me into a wall and Dave told me no one would love me like him (since I had cancer). Should I have done the work to improve myself before getting back out into the world of dating? Should I have gone to counseling and healed myself and talked to someone and figured out how to get past Dave telling me I *had a weird vagina?*

Absolutely, I should have.

I just felt like I didn't have time.

I had brain cancer.

There was a global pandemic.

I had someone in front of me who, despite a few weird

missteps and pretending to be a werewolf on a Google phone number, was making interesting enough conversation and keeping me company after an MRI, which, despite the fantastic night I had with Josh, he sure wasn't doing.

I wanted to prove I still had it in me, prove I could still, after being diagnosed with brain cancer, seduce a stranger into coming up to my hotel room, which, funny enough, I was very against doing two nights before.

Well, are you ready to get out of here? Timmatthew asks as he checks his phone again. Is that a text message? It is. It's not his precious ponies.

I am! Let me pay. It was your birthday recently.

Aw, no, I can't let you do that.

I want to impress him with the knowledge I remembered his birthday, and no, I didn't snoop around and find it like the *crazy women* he mentioned, but he told me in a text, and despite my brain issues, I didn't forget.

The bartender gives Timmatthew the tab.

I only had three gin-and-tonics, but it feels like I had 12.

Is his name Tim or Matthew? After someone lies to you about something as basic as their name, the truth becomes as opaque as my gin-and-tonic hotel glass.

How many heartbreaks in this bar, I wonder?

We walk toward the elevator, and this time will be different. I will get into the elevator and recognize the person standing beside me. Timmatthew will tell me how he's been waiting for this first date to happens so he can express his feelings for me. We have been texting for a couple months now. I've told him about Josh, hoping to get him to move off the ledge, so I'm assuming this will be the night he does it. He just needed the alcohol to soften his feelings up a bit, and once we are in the hotel room, he will go for it and express his love.

Sure, I had a magical night with Josh, but it was a glittery glitch in my relationship matrix that needed to happen to clear the way for other paths. Sure, there were a few odd moments in my conversation with Timmathew and some glances at his cell phone (mine was put away the whole time), but I want to give this a chance. Sure, there was the whole catfishing thing, but I've put that behind me like a bad line, I'm ready to move forward and see where this potential relationship goes.

We get to the elevator doors, and I press the up button.

I turn toward him to make a joke or say something dumb and charming.

Thanks for meeting up, he says as he gives me a quick hug. *See you later*.

The elevator opens, and I stand there as he walks toward the hotel exit.

Are ya fucking kidding me?

After months of sexting and texting and getting to know one another, I thought this was a sure thing. I *knew* this was a sure thing. Who would put so much effort into getting to know me, spend an hour having drinks with me, and then bounce like absolutely nothing happened? Didn't he at least want to test the chemistry and make out?

There had been a lot of buildup, after all.

The last time I felt this confident about something was when the surgeon walked into my hospital room. I thought for sure he would say, *Congrats! It's a benign tumor!* and instead he said, *Unfortunately* and the hospital tiles disappeared from underneath my paralyzed foot.

It's a dramatic comparison, but the feeling is slightly reminiscent.

I did not expect to get rejected like this.

The elevator door shuts, and I am humiliated I didn't get inside.

I press the button again; I need to make it up to my room

and order some fucking Bojangles or something to eat my sadness away.

I can't believe this shit.

When I finally make it into the elevator, I open DoorDash on my phone. I need to eat to counteract this alcohol. I remember someone telling me that like Huntington, the Bojangles in Charleston closed, so I'm going to have to go another route.

I find some kind of spaghetti, and I plan to get real messy and makes sure it gets all over my face. No one will be there to see the shit I'm about to do, and it's going to be bad.

The tears come in the hallway. I'm drunker than I thought and can barely walk. Did I ever press the order button for DoorDash?

Fuck.

I text Josh.

I had a bad date.

I leave out the part that it's bad because Timmatthew rejected me by not coming to my room like I planned.

I am drunk enough to go for the dreaded double text, the thing I keep saying I never do.

It was a bad date because it wasn't with you.

Josh replies right away, which tells me he was with his phone all day and could have texted me if he wanted to but didn't.

I'm sorry you had a bad date.

Excuse me?

I'm sorry you had a bad date?

That's all he has to say?

I'm out here looking for the one I'm supposed to be with, and everyone is turning out to be a dead, floppy fish. Fight for me, Josh, I want to tell him. Say *It should have been me. It would have been way better* or *Make it me next time, and we will have as much fun as we did the other night.*

I stop myself. Maybe I'm asking for too much.

No.

I told Josh I was dating other people, but was open, very open, very very open, to something with him. Timmatthew, since I met him online, was obviously following the protocol of everyone else online dating and also seeing other people but not talking about it to the billion other people he was dating.

I was doing nothing wrong by wanting someone to step up. I had also expressed to anyone and everyone how I was looking to spend the rest of my *dying days*—even if I happened to only have 12 or 30 or 17 or 52— with one person and was tired of fucking around with all of this casual dating bullshit.

Once in my room, which I'm surprised I found, I begin to suspect the problem is me. How could it not be? Something about me, Suzanne Samples, is driving these people away. Men. Women. Friends. I've lost them all. It can't be the brain cancer, but that might have something to do with it.

It's me.

It has to be.

In the depths of my gin-and-tonic self-pity, something changes.

My phone buzzes, and I feel hopeful.

Maybe it's Timmatthew saying he's still outside the hotel, waiting for me to invite him up, romantic comedy style.

Maybe it's Josh saying he's driving to Charleston because he wants to see me one more time before I go back to Harrisville.

Hey! It's Anna, your DoorDash driver. It turns out the restaurant is out of the garlic aioli you ordered with your spaghetti. Is there another sauce you would like?

Oh, my fucking god.

166

This is not Anna's fault this is not Anna's fault this is not Anna's fault.

Meat sauce on the side is fine! Thanks so much.

I go into the bathroom and sit on the toilet. My left side, my good side, feels completely numb. *This can't be happening it's just because I'm drunk nooooo it can't be.* I can't move either of my legs. Fucking gin-and-tonics. Fucking Timmatthew. Fucking Josh. I sit there frozen. Although I desperately have to pee, my bladder won't work. My body feels paralyzed from my hips down. It's just the alcohol. It has to be. I take a few deep breaths and consider jumping into the shower and washing the day off of me, but I can't.

I. Can't. Move.

I imagine someone finding me like this. Somehow my clothes came off before I got on the toilet. It's better this way, Timmatthew not coming up. What a shit show this would have been. My god, what is happening? I place my hands on the bathroom tile and slowly disintegrate into the floor. This is the perk of paying for an upscale hotel. I don't have to worry about falling into absolute filth.

I have a seizure on the clean tiles.

This, however, causes me no alarm.

It feels good to move.

This is my own fault; I shouldn't have had so much to drink. Three cocktails wouldn't bother most people, but as I've heard from other brain tumor patients, tolerance goes way down after experiencing a tumor or surgery.

I feel like I've had more drinks and drugs than a coked-out rock star.

I am shaking shaking shaking from the seizure, but I stay awake. I always do, thankfully.

When Anna knocks at the door with my spaghetti, I think

about calling to her and asking if she will bust through and help me up.

I feel like such a loser.

It's no wonder no one wants to be with me.

The floor is cold, the towels are too excitable here.[11]

I use the towels as kneepads like I did in my roller derby days and the toilet as a ledge to steady myself as I stand. The seizure seems to have bested the numbness in both legs, and although I'm still drunk, I can stand and almost kind of walk.

I grab the spare key so I don't lock myself out and grab the DoorDash bag from the hallway. Thank you, Anna. I will leave you a stellar review, my friend. My only friend. I open the curtain and gaze at the Charleston night sky. Although I'm expecting a cityscape, all I see are a few stray bulbs aglow in a damp, dull night.

Welcome to Charleston.

I inhale the spaghetti and don't even look to see how much I got on my face, though I'm sure it's most of it.

I'm like a child.

I eat the middle out of some garlic bread and crack open a Coke. I don't give any insulin. Why would it matter? No one is checking on me. Everyone assumes I *am strong enough to do this on my own.* I keep checking my phone to see if any messages have arrived, but there is nothing.

Not a thing.

Not a single person has thought of me, except this spaghetti.

I am confused.

Although I'm sure this portion is for a large man, I finish the entire meal, Coke, and all. This should send my blood sugar to a level reaching the top floor of the hotel, but I don't care. Who would even know at this point?

Not a soul.

Somewhere in the middle of all this, everything in my mind goes terribly wrong. I don't know how I ended up here in Charleston, West Virginia, alone in a hotel room, drunk on gin and tonic and full of spaghetti.

I open Tinder.

I match with a guy name James and message him with interest. He lives in Charleston, and I figure, what the hell? I can take a quick shower, brush my teeth, and invite him over for a one-night stand.

Really not my style but neither is cancer.

Me: *Hey! Whatcha up to tonight?*

James: *Not much hot t. Just in town for work. U?*

Ugh, the letters instead of actual words make me shiver with disgust. Or maybe it's another seizure. Hard to say at this point.

Me: *The same, actually. What do you do for a living?*

Him: *Construction. U?*

One night one night I can do this one night one night one night.

Me: *I'm an English teacher. I'm here for a conference. One night only.*

Sure, why not.

Him: *Suzanne's a pretty name. Where do you teach.*

Okay, I'm naïve sometimes. I assume he wants to get to know me a bit before he comes over. I don't assume he's stalking me on social media.

Me: *I teach English at a school called Appalachian State University. To be frank, I'm just looking to hook up for the night.*

He doesn't answer. I'm confused; I thought this was the ultimate dream of all men on Tinder: no strings attached hookups.

Him: *Ur hot and all but sorry I can't hook up with a Nazi.*

A Nazi? Nothing about my Tinder profile or this conversa-

169

tion would ever lead anyone to believe I'm anything close to a Nazi.

And then I understand; Suzanne is not a super common name. Even if James cannot write a complete sentence, he can Google Suzanne+Appalachian State+English, find my last name, search my Facebook page, and see my formerly bald head from the damn brain cancer.

Jesus.

Me: I HAVE FUCKING CANCER, YOU ASSHOLE.

And then it's over. I lose it. I've had a-fucking-nough of everyone. I don't understand why I have to deal with any of this bullshit. I don't understand why I have brain cancer. I get it—it could be worse, babies in African countries have cancer and don't get treatment at all, blah blah blah, but I just need a moment here to pity myself, which to be honest, I haven't had. It's been go go go since I was diagnosed. Relearn to walk. Radiation. Chemo. Appointments. Telling everyone I AM OKAY. Yes, I have brain cancer, but I am okay. I. Am. Okay. I am okay I am okay I am okay, everyone! Smile. Repeat. Smile! Yes, I am really fucking okay, I swear. I swear! I'm just driving my parents from appointment to appointment and waiting and waiting on them and grading papers my students don't care about and think are dumb and I'm putting so much time into this and getting paid pennies, pure pennies for meticulously poring over each and every word Ashlynn and Sydneigh and Kylynn and Braxley pay someone else to write, but everything is fine. Everything is fine! I fucking promise! I just keep going from MRI to appointments and swallowing these pills and puking and acting like I'm going to be fine while losing most of my friends and relationships and my teeth (and paying thousands of dollars to get them replaced) and talking to these guys on Tinder who want to get me drunk but won't even make out with me and think I'm a Nazi but I. Am. Fucking. Fine. I promise.

Really.

Except that I'm not at all.

Not even close.

I am mentally crashing hard.

I dig through my piles on the floor. Whenever I travel, it looks as if I threw a grenade in my bag and stuff just explodes everywhere. I don't know why I do this. I've always been this way, and now that I'm pushing 40, I don't think I'll change.

I find a mega bottle of ibuprofen PM and about 16.5 Klonopin I have for emergencies.

Well, this seems like an emergency.

I dump every pill onto the hotel desk and search for water. I'm not baller enough to swallow them dry. I fill up a smudged hotel glass and start with the ibuprofen PMs.

One.

Two.

Three.

Four.

Five.

I take a break and line up all 16.5 Klonopin on the desk.

One.

Two.

I want to do this on my own terms. My way. I want to separate from my brain, since it has decided to do its own damn thing, and just do it this way instead. Forget the cancer bullshit.

And then I stop.

I don't want a cleaning lady or man to find me. That would be some fucked up shit they do not get paid enough for. What am I doing? I can't do this to someone who gets paid minimum wage. If I don't care about myself, I at least care about people who don't get paid enough to find a dead body.

I message about seven people I know who have brain cancer.

Hey, is anyone up?

Ugh, this is a bad idea; it's late. Too late. These people I'm messaging have kids, families. Responsibilities. I shouldn't have done any of this. I am embarrassed, ashamed. At least if I'm messaging other people with cancer, they will have some idea why I'm upset, why I'm suicidal. I feel like if I message anyone else, nothing will make any sense.

I pull myself together and search *suicide hotline for cancer patients.*

Thank you for your search. Our hotline is run by volunteers and open from 9 a.m. to 8 p.m. on weekdays.

Jesus Christ, Fog Woman, Hindu Floaty Thingy.

I want to take the entire bottle of K-pins and call it a night. A week. A lifetime.

My big question: What, exactly, was the point of getting through all *this?*

This.

A euphemism for brain surgery, radiation, chemo, staying up late every night, dreaming of dying, people having no idea what to say to me, feeling like I have zero support from people who were supposed to care for me the most, moving home and thinking my parents were going to take care of me when it turned out I was taking care of them and losing my goddamn mind from it, constantly wondering if my cancer was back, working to ensure this hemiparesis didn't ruin the rest of whatever life I had left, friends never returning my texts, feeling isolated, trying to lose this forever limp leg, Tinder dates acting like they are interested when they really aren't at all, stretching a magical night with an old fling into something just a little bit longer, and then, finally, being called a Nazi and spreading a bunch of pills out onto a hotel desk and taking as many as I could before realizing maybe, just maybe, I should talk to someone about this first.

Fuck it.

I am scared of what I might do.

I am worried and concerned for my safety.

I call the good ol' general suicide hotline.

A voice answers. The voice of a mother. I don't know if she's actually a mother, but she sounds like one. I give her my trust like I'm handing her the most fragile, infant bird.

Hey, baby. Tell me exactly what's going on.

She's the kind of woman who can call you *baby*, and it doesn't seem weird or abnormal. Her words are like a warm cup of apple cider.

I have cancer, and I'm in a hotel after an MRI, and I don't know the results, and I just don't want to do this anymore. I'm young, and it's a weird cancer that people don't really seem to understand. It's gone but not really. I don't even know if I understand it myself. It's just—and then my mom had a stroke and I had to move and take care of her, and my dad—he's sick too and they rely on me and I just can't do it. I need help. I just can't keep going on like this. And I'm lonely and want to—

Okay, just take a couple breaths. This is hard stuff. Do people actually try to make you feel like this is easy? Because that's just stupid!

I laugh.

I still feel like dying, but I laugh.

They do try to make me feel like this is easy. I'm a really strong person, but I just can't do all this stuff all the time. It's too much, and I just want it to end. I just can't do it. I feel like ending it all the time, and I'm not kidding. Despite my strength, though, I just don't feel like I'm strong enough to actually go through with it.

Do you want to tell me more about that?

173

I do want to tell her more about that.

I know the number of pills I took won't actually do anything but knock me out really well, which I probably need. I tell her how lonely I am, how despite having people around me all the time, they just seem to want to take take take from me without ever wanting to actually support me or love me for who I am. Sure, people like Josh will hear my story and catch up with me for an evening, but past that? It's too much.

She just listens.

I talk to this stranger until 2 a.m., and you know what? She helps me. She really does. I ramble and I cry and I tell her *I don't really want to die, but it seems better to die from killing myself than it does from brain cancer.* She doesn't claim to know or understand or suggest I should extract the latent juices from a peach pit to cure everything.

She just listens.

I tell her about my mom and my dad and how I do my best to care for them but it's too much, and I feel like I may have been manipulated into this whole thing and now I can't get out of it.

She just listens.

I tell her how I'm romantically isolated and keep trying to meet someone, but I just got rejected and then called a Nazi, and it's not true, not true at all, and she laughs out of horror and so do I, and then we are both laughing because the whole thing is so ridiculous, and I think we both know, even though she's only known me for maybe an hour now, I can do better than this. I play with my hair that's grown back quite a bit, and I wonder if I'll ever be good enough for anyone, and the stranger on the phone reads my mind and says, *Girl, don't stoop to some stupid man's level like that ever again. Don't let other people, people you don't even know, determine how you feel about your-*

self, and I feel like this free advice is worth more than I could ever receive in hundreds of dollars of professional counseling.

Before we hang up, she tells me I should hug both my parents when I get home, and I tell her my family *isn't the hugging type,* and she says, *Surprise them! Do it anyway!* and I think I just might.

When I wake up the next morning, I'm alive but my blood sugar is somehow 39, a dangerously low level. I Uber Eats some Starbucks, scarf it down, and stare at the pills still lined up on the table like forgotten soldiers, all lonelier than I was the night before.

Harrisville, West Virginia

I get home and change my clothes. No one asks how I'm feeling (hungover) or how everything went.

There is no hugging, but it was a nice thought.

I've learned no one, not even my parents, care how my MRI went. If they do, they don't show it. I know everyone could offer hundreds of excuses. *You're just so independent. They don't want to step on your toes. They think you can handle this on your own.*

Last evening shows I clearly cannot, but I don't know where to turn.

I get it's a complicated situation. No one knows what to do with me. I'm in this weird space where I don't really have active cancer; it's just planted there in my head like a weed waiting to bloom again. I haven't processed the trauma from the shocking surgery, chemo, and radiation yet, but I'm looking for someone to accept me as I am, and all I can find are boys who want to breadcrumb me.

So, I do what anyone in my situation would and purchase a

few ghost hunting items from Amazon and prepare myself to discover more about the unknown.

I lace up my boots and head to the cemetery to commune with the dead. I don't want to sit in this house and think about what happened last night. I'm somewhere between embarrassingly horrified and the saddest I've ever been, and I'd rather spend some time with people who have nothing to say, rather than hear my dad talk about the weather and my mom discuss church.

I wish Amazon drones delivered ghost hunting equipment to rural West Virginia.

I also need to walk off the spaghetti I devoured last night, thanks to Anna.

I'm grateful there is no one at the cemetery, except the people who can't leave. I abandon the track to peruse all the old crumbling gravesites and silently beg them for guidance. *What happens to us? Where do we end up? Tell me, Ulyssus Moats. Damn, you were only 15. I feel like an asshole complaining to you.* I wish I had my paranormal equipment already so I could afford better communication with Ulyssus.

My phone vibrates.

How are ya?

Josh.

Really?

Nothing and then my *bad date* but then we are just going to pretend that didn't happen and start over.

My phone buzzes again.

The ponies won me some money today!

Timmatthew.

I stand in the grass and consider what I'm missing here. These guys don't really want to be with me, but they want my attention? Why? I don't understand. I'm losing interest in games I don't know I'm playing.

I decide to walk it off.

Everything.

The MRI I don't know the results of and won't until next week. The mixed messages from everyone in my life. (We care! We don't care! We want you around! We don't! Wait, we want you around, but only when we have time for you!) When I've jaunted five miles around the track and talked with Ulyssus, I feel much better.

After I greet my parents when I get home, I download Bumble, which gives women the power to reach out first, and as Betsy tells me, *is for more serious daters.*

I want to be a more serious dater.

I am done messing around.

I want someone real.

I see Damien's profile right away. He's a ginger-blond who lives somewhere in Ohio (everywhere around here is rural, so there's that) and works in "Travel." I'm not exactly sure what that means—it could be anything from a travel agent to a couch surfer, and I'm honestly afraid to ask.

I take my chances.

We have similar taste in music, down to the album, so I write a thesis concerning Nathaniel Rateliff and Marlon Williams—it's seriously a three-paragraph long hello—and press send. Feeling sassy, I end with, "And how's that for an opener?"

I think I've struck indie gold.

If it was anyone other than Damien, I might have been reported because the opener is a bit intense. Not inappropriate but intense. It's a far cry from *Hey!* or *Hi, how are you?* or the ever popular *wyd?*

He doesn't seem to mind.

Damien wants to add me on Snapchat and write to me about all the ice cream he's eaten this evening, which I should have taken as a sign we would never meet. We briefly discuss getting together but send each other dirty pics instead. What's the harm? I'm going to die anyway. Single, probably. I might as well have some fun.

Perhaps I should rethink the entire Bumble shebang.

One evening Damien gets excited and says, *I'm going to send you a newd (a brand new one!),* and then texts the same one he Snapped three weeks ago, a black-and-white artsy number with weed smoke trailing above his privates like ribbon dancers at a music festival. I think he is really high, so I forgive him. My sister and I call him *Dirty Dabs Damien,* but in a loving way.

He's fun and harmless, but this doesn't absolve my loneliness.[12]

Ellenboro, West Virginia, the Dick Bias Tunnel, Tunnel #10, 377 ft.

I'm guessing The Dick Bias Tunnel is the most popular tunnel on the trail. I have no proof of this, but it's easily accessible and by far, the most beautiful. To make the tunnel, builders bored straight into solid rock and made a 377-foot corridor. It's the only all-natural tunnel on the trail, and on humid West Virginia summer days, the passageway feels refreshing and not creepy like the others.

Dick Bias was a cool guy, my dad says, and if Mr. Samples says Dick Bias was cool, he must have been a helluva person.

Sometimes I like to stop in this tunnel and chill when I'm walking the trail. It's non-threatening; the sunlight gets in, but the heat doesn't. I like to touch the cool, wet stones and imagine how many hikers and bikers have journeyed through this small town in search of something.

We are all in search of something.

Although people pierced through natural rock to create this work of art, the builders did a bang-up job of making the tunnel look like it happened out of nowhere. The way the rocks jut out toward the trail and into the passageway of the tunnel present a fun challenge for bikers going a bit too fast, but there's still no need to turn on a headlamp or feel frightened.

This is a safe space.

A natural place in the hills of West Virginia, maybe not meant to be here, but one certainly not doing any harm to the scenery like the fracking down the road.

I spend a lot of time in this tunnel. For one, it's excellent practice. There's just enough darkness to check my balance but still plenty of light to make it easy to see my surroundings.

I feel at peace here.

At any moment, a chipmunk or squirrel might join me on the trail.

However, I must keep moving.

I need to keep walking, and these tunnels are meant to be part of a voyage.

Harrisville, West Virginia

My doctor looks small and lonely and faraway on the Zoom screen.

We lost your scans, but I finally called Charleston and got a copy, he says.

Someone must have dumped them in the Kanawha River, I joke, but no one laughs.

I hold my breath. Why is no one laughing?

Congrats! Another boring MRI! Same as last time.

I exhale but know this can't last forever.

PART III
GHOSTS

Cairo/Cornwallis, West Virginia, Tunnels #13 & 12

On a random Tuesday, Josh wants to visit me in Harrisville.

Although I'm extremely confused, I figure why not?

He offers to *do anything, go anywhere I want to go* that afternoon. He's going to drive from Huntington to Harrisville, which is about two-and-a-half hours one way, meet me, take me anywhere, then go back to work that night.

This is the most Josh thing ever.

Of course, we can't really *do anything, go anywhere*, so I suggest the tunnels. He brings his camera, and we take off to North Bend.

I've never shared these tunnels with anyone outside of Harrisville, and I am curious what he will think.

We don't talk much on the way there, but it's a comfortable silence. I mention my hand hurting, which I fear is a sign *my cancer is back.*

I'll learn later I'm exactly right.

When we get to the tunnels, Josh prepares his camera equipment, and I'm in awe of everything he has: lenses, tripods, and frames I can't name. He bends down and asks me to *put his hair up in a bun,* and I comply.

We've always been this comfortable.

Josh and I walk toward the tunnels, and I feel myself relaxing about everything: the MRIs, the need to be in a relationship, living at home with my parents, everything. With Josh, I have manifested this ability to think less and live more.

The tunnels look extra horror-movie ready tonight, and Josh sets up his camera. I observe him, as if he will be the first one picked off, but we all know I'm the one in danger. He snaps a few pics, and I remember why I have always loved Josh so much.

Because it will never work out.

Fog sets in, making the tunnels look endless and extra spooky. Josh and I walk back toward his car on the dark trail, and we decide to eat in the state park's Twin Peaks[1]-esque restaurant. I've never eaten here without my grandparents and not on a Sunday after church.

The waitress somehow knows me and also assumes Josh and I are married. *Just go with it,* I tell him, and we laugh. We order some sort of mashed potato special that the server assures us was *better in the afternoon,* and I can't finish mine, so Josh does.

Y'all have kids yet? the waitress asks, and I explode into gravy giggles.

No. Not really our thing.

Good for you. I have three and regret it all the time. She takes a beat as she pours us more iced tea. *I mean, not really, but ya know. Tell Mr. Samples I said hi.*

Will do.

Later, I'll tell my dad *a girl who works at the park said hi. Short. Younger than me. Dark hair,* and he will say, *Oh, yeah, that's Rachel. She's a nice girl.*

Unknowingly, the waitress helps me segue into talking to Josh about relationships, and before I know it, I'm no longer living in the moment! Free! Not thinking! but doing the opposite. I put some pressure on Josh and ask how he feels about them.

Relationships.

Monogamous relationships, open relationships, any sort of relationships, really. I think this should be enough to clue Josh in that perhaps, I want a relationship with him, but he doesn't follow my train of thought.

Once we return to his car, we can't keep our hands off each other, though, so he pulls off a side road, and we try to mess around, but we become cliched deer in headlights when a truck pulls towards us.

I know another place we can go, I say, and I direct him back toward Harrisville.

No one will be at the cemetery; it's nice and dark and the Ulyssus won't care what Josh and I do.

Morbid, Josh says, *but okay.*

We drive there in silence, except for Josh saying he *feels like a teenager* and me giving directions.

After parking the car, Josh rips his pants off.

I take off my shirt.

A few minutes later, the cemetery lights up, as if we've skipped the mountain night completely and gone straight to morning on a hot beach somewhere.

The fuck? Josh says, feeling quite alarmed but too dazed to pull up his pants. *Cops!*

Everything is visible in his vehicle, down to the last dust particle.

I know exactly what is happening.

Dammit.

It's not cops. I forgot about the giant, slowly rotating cross-

185

of-Jesus beacon that turns on around 7 p.m. every evening at the graveyard. The damn thing must be 30-feet tall, and you can see it from anywhere in town.

We parked directly under the old rugged cross, and Jesus has seen everything, and I mean everything. Josh and I are naked under the eyes of Christ himself, and if anyone were to drive up here at this moment, they would get quite a show.

Josh and I explode into laughter.

It's like being in high school again, he says.

I know, I reply, and he has no idea how right he is, the lightbulbs of Jesus turning in unison above us, judging our every move.

He told me later the pictures didn't turn out; something, he's not sure what, was wrong with the film.

Harrisville, West Virginia

My paranormal equipment has arrived.

I have been studying and watching many YouTube videos regarding how to commune with the dead respectfully.

I start to think these tunnels probably have a lot to offer. I don't want to put anything on YouTube or become a famous, monetized blogger, but I want answers.

I want to know what lies beyond the limits of what we see and experience daily, and I think these tunnels know. Naturally, I have selfish reasons for all this. It's not strange for me to question what might happen after death. I've come close, and I might never be too far away. At any moment, this brain cancer could return and multiply as quickly as I go exploring through those structures.

I want to know what's on the other side.

I want to see.

I want to hear.

I want to experience the unknown and come back before I stay forever.

I want to see the other side. I know I will be there soon, and I want to understand what it's like. I want to feel less scared. I want to get a glimpse of what might happen when I'm gone.

I have no doubt people like my mom will go to heaven. I'm of the mindset that whatever you believe, you will become. If my mom wants the streets of gold and to sit at the right hand of God, she will do so. But what about people like me who just aren't sure? There could be something out there, but I just don't know.

I need to see it for myself.

Now I just need to figure out how.

I bought an EMF reader, a digital voice recorder, and a spirit box. Theoretically, the EMF reader will tell me where the spirits are. I can hopefully use the spirit box (which is a radio with a button used for quick skipping to catch *electric voice phenomenon*, or little blips between the airways that create words like *help* or names calling from the grave), and then catch all of this with the digital recorder.

Okay, I need more hands.

Especially if I plan to do this in a dark tunnel.

I start sleeping with the spirit box near my bed because I read it needs to *attach itself* to me. I am not against this, but I am scared it might cause something fearful to happen to my family. To be honest, I don't care so much about myself at this point. If some evil dark force grabs hold of me, then I don't feel like I have much to lose.

I want spirits to find me.

To reach me.

To speak to me.

Although I don't want to fuck up my parents' new house, I can't avoid the temptation of using the spirit box and EMF reader in my bedroom. I scan the airways and hear nothing but some old AM stations, which does take me back to my childhood. I scan faster and faster and think I hear a blip of *hey hey hey*, but I convince myself I am imagining things, or maybe a station is playing The Lumineers. I walk around my new little space in the house and notice the EMF reader lights up when near microwaves and other electronic equipment.

Lesson learned: just because a tree lights up doesn't mean it's Christmas.

With hope renewed, I decide to return to the Clarksburg area tomorrow and search the area with my new equipment. If I don't find the tunnels, hopefully I will find something.

Anything.

Anyone.

I wonder if people have committed suicide in these tunnels. It's a dark thought, but one worth considering. I fantasize I might be the one to free a spirit from being trapped in there. It's not out of the question. With all of the trains coming through this area, there might have been tons of people jumping in front of them. If people had been waiting in the tunnels, the conductors would have never seen them, and then it would have been too late to do anything about it.

How fucking sad.

But for now, I need to find this Brandy Gap Tunnel, for real this time, and check it off the list.

I take the EMF reader and spirit box but not the recorder.

I jump back in the tiny Scion and head to the Clarksburg area to find this damn tunnel. I search different GPS coordinates this time, and somehow end up at the Harrison Power Station. The building seems innocuous, but I know better: Power plants mean the formation of creatures like The Mothman, and then nothing is the same ever again.

Three identical coal chimneys—the father, son, and the

holy spirit— beckon to me, and I feel like I'm in the show *Dark*. If there's a tunnel here, there's definitely a God particle somewhere inside of it, and I'm traveling somewhere backward or forward in time. It all fits: small town, people having all sorts of affairs, now all we need are some kids disappearing and some weird experiments happening in the 1980s with some red, neon wallpaper, and then we will be headed toward an apocalypse in three days.

I wander around the outskirts of the powerplant and wait for someone to ask for a badge or something, but no one does. I walk around like I own the place, and no one says a word.

I spot a box where it seems an employee might sit.

I don't really have an accent, but like a medium at a séance sponsored by pepperoni rolls, I can surely conjure one up to increase my credibility—*Do y'all know where that tunnel is?*

But no one is there.

Does anyone work here at all?

I decide to search for a trail; it's got to be near here.

I walk for a minute.

There is nothing but open air.

Polluted open air.

I finally walk long enough to find a patch of dirt that sort of resembles a trailhead, but who the fuck would put a trailhead near a power plant?

West Virginia would.

I've already exercised a fair amount and am a bit tired. I don't know where this trail goes, and although I'm not far from home, I'm too far to know anyone or for anyone to know me. There's a familiarity in the areas where my mom has worked or my dad has taught school, and I'm too far from the periphery now.

Defeated, I turn back.

I'll find the tunnel later.

. . .

Charleston/Huntington, West Virginia

I fall into a bizarre pattern of visiting Josh in Huntington and Timmatthew in Charleston on the way home. Josh fulfills my need for love and companionship, while Timmatthew fulfills the need for desire.

I want either of them to fulfill both, but this doesn't seem to happen.

During a visit to a coffee shop in Huntington, Josh offhandedly tells me he *wants to be more monk-like in the coming days.* He wants to concentrate more on his art and have nothing to do with sex or relationships.

I'm a bit stunned and don't know what to think.

Before this, I assumed we were moving in the direction of a relationship. I was visiting frequently, meeting more of his friends, sleeping in his bed, and of course, we were hooking up. I drink my iced coffee and tell myself to *not get upset. This is Josh. He may change his mind an hour later.* He tells me he loves me when we part ways that day, and I say the same in return.

I am headed to Betsy's house, but first, I drive around old Huntington, where I used to live. I have a long talk with myself. Yes, I love Josh, but do I really want to be with someone who is going to look me straight in the eye and tell me that although we've been hanging out and hooking up and declaring our love for one another, he all of the sudden wants to be more like a monk now? I've done far too much work on my personal life to hang onto some weird romantic aspirations for someone to tell me he wants to *be like a monk.*

Without realizing, I have pulled onto the brick streets of Jefferson Avenue, where I lived when I first met Josh. I am in front of the same apartment where we climbed into the window after coming in from the V Club, slightly drunk and wondering what the night would bring.

I let Josh go then and there.

We will always be friends.

I know this.

At Betsy's, my Tinder nightmares make good stories for her and her new husband. They give me a new perspective, and I feel refreshed. We make dinner reservations and stop at Empire Books beforehand. I am delighted to see they have *Frontal Matter* on their shelves and take a quick picture when no one is looking. When I was an English major at Marshall, I never dreamed I would walk into the bookstore here and see my actual name on an actual book. The world feels surreal, or maybe it's just the margarita I had earlier.

Late into the night, I get a text and can't sleep.

It's Timmatthew.

I have no idea what I'm doing, but it's not good.

Why are you in Huntington? Come to Charleston.

I tell him no, but we both can see in the crystal ball of our cell phones that I'm eventually going to acquiesce. I leave Betsy a note and sneak out. I feel a little badly about this, but I think they will understand.

Betsy knows how much I want to find a relationship.

Betsy also knows, better than I do, how this is nothing more than a booty call for Timmatthew.

When I show up at his house, he's asleep. I call call call him, and I wonder if he's ever going to answer. I recall a story Betsy just told me about a sex worker who recently ended up deceased in a trash can.

Answer your fucking phone, I implore.

Finally, he shows up at the door and leads me upstairs.

* * *

191

I wake up the big spoon.

You're going to hate me, Timmatthew says, *but my girls are coming over. You have to go.*

I am more than happy to go.

I just want to brush my teeth.

I make myself at home in the guest bathroom, brush my teeth, and try to pee, but I'm too nervous. About what, I'm not sure.

When I struggle down the stairs, I see Timmatthew furiously setting up a tea party for his twins. This endears him to me, and I forget about what an asshole he is sometimes. I remind myself: People are rarely bad or good but always on a spectrum of qualities at any given time, myself included.

Give me a hug, I demand as I give him a copy of my book, I signed in his guest bathroom. This is the last time I will ever see him, but he *will* remember Suzanne Samples. He halfheartedly hugs me then opens the door.

I disappear into the gray of Charleston, knowing it is forever going to be this way.

Cairo, West Virginia, Tunnel # 17, 452 feet

There's something so forgotten about these tunnels and trails that bothers me. Why does no one talk about them? Why does hardly anyone care about them? Why doesn't anyone understand just how interesting and fascinating they are?

I've discovered so much about myself in these tunnels.

Who I am now.

(Am I required to be anything at all? I don't think so.)

Who I am supposed to be, if anyone.

(I am enjoying being nothing most of the time.)

After surgery and my cancer diagnosis, I lost everything.

(Was anything I thought I had so important? Looking back, I see it wasn't so much of anything.)

I reimagined myself here in these open-ended caves.

Found myself again.

Walking through these structures in the dark, I didn't know what I would find; to anyone else, it may have sounded like a bunch of dripping and smelled of moldy memories of forgotten people and once-thriving towns, but now the tunnels sit and wait for me to read them, to investigate them, to share them with you.

I like the tunnels that have been bypassed by the trails, as if they have been forgotten by everyone and left aside to rot.

Number 17 is one of those tunnels.

I have walked past this tunnel probably seven or eight times while exercising on the trail and failed to notice the beast. How do you miss a giant stone train tunnel? Quite easy to do when the entire entity is overgrown with muddy green moss and covered in last autumn's leaves. It seems to just disappear within the woods, which adds to its mystique.

The dark, damp day adds to the mystery of #17. Although people from my hometown might have their own stories, I currently don't know of any from this particular tunnel, but I get a strange feeling before I cut from the path and enter.

I don't turn on my headlamp; something tells me not to. I want to sink into this darkness and let the stillness speak to me as only it can. Light cannot teach me, only darkness. Since what I've been through, I've realized happiness has only small gifts to offer, and as a person, I don't thrive in the light. Of course, I smile and am at peace and love people and am grateful for what life has given me.

But really?

I am a creature who thrives in this in between, this bleakness, these words no one wants to write. This tunnel is my home, and if I fall, I will find protection in the nameless spirits of those who came before me and felt the same way.

I could live in this tunnel, #17, although it's not my favorite (which would be #12), but still, I could stay here for as long as necessary. I stand for a moment past the entry so I am ensconced by dripping blackness. I was never a goth kid or Wiccan, but just someone who went and continues to go my own way. I lean against the tunnel wall, not caring how wet I get or what my parents will say to me.

I scan through the spirit box. I have been sleeping with it, so I hope the contraption has attached itself to me like an old friend or companion pet. Nothing on the FM, but I have a feeling AM will be a better bet. The tunnel is as silent as a mausoleum, and I wish for a memorial bench in here for all the ones we have lost.

Instead, I sit in one of my familiar alcoves, which are all relatively the same. I look like a forgotten lover lonely in the dark, not a young adult with cancer trying to find some sort of ghosts who passed through this town long ago. I put my spirit box on autoscan, and while I'm sitting in the lantern spot, I start to hear a brief whisper.

Suz.

Suz.

Suz.

I swear my imagination is creating these syllables, but it's there *Suz Suz Suz.* What my sister calls me. For a brief moment, this brain cancer shit seems worth it.

I have connected to the other side.

Something grander than myself.

The surgery, the loss of my right foot, the paralysis, the betrayal of friends, the misery the misery the misery.

Someone has something to say to me.

The spiritbox continues to autoscan, but the clarity of *Suz* is gone.

In my haste, I drop the spiritbox to look for the EMF reader to see if I'm in a preeminent spot for any other voices who might need to speak to me. I find the EMF reader, and it scans yellow, which means fine, I'm in an okay spot, unless there is a hidden microwave or other electronic device somewhere in this tunnel.

There's definitely something here, an entity of sorts, but I'm unsure if this tunnel spirit is *good* or *bad*.

Spirits seem to fall into these black and white categories. When I imagine myself as an entity, though, it's difficult to believe I would fall into such a distinction.

Naturally, plenty of evidence exists of bad spirits; from Zozo on the Ouija Board to demonic possessions in Catholicism, no one wants these guys around, but I don't feel like they are hanging out in the North Bend State Park Rail Trail Tunnels. Even the suicidal track hoppers couldn't be evil—they were all just trying to escape something.

Weren't we all just trying to escape something?

I do know one thing for sure: I do not feel scared.

The spirit of Tunnel #17 feels protective.

Even if a bad spirit would chase me, I don't feel they would get very far.

The EMF reader flicks from yellow to green.

I have renewed hope I am not alone.

Even if I cannot touch this entity, I want to feel something here with me now.

Although it's on the muddy ground, the spiritbox still scans, but all I hear are frequencies not meant for me. I stay seated and wait.

Sometimes patience is needed.

I have learned this.

Patience in hospitals.

Patience in diagnoses.

Patience on radiation tables.

Patience with the ending of puking.

Patience patience patience.

Patience with writing.

I wait for the spirits to speak to me. It's likely just residual energy, echoes of souls who won't go away. I have a feeling I'll be like this, and I hate myself for it already. I will just refuse to leave, refuse to disappear, and annoy everyone forever.

Maybe I just need to sit here longer.

The spirit box dies, and the light on my headlamp dims. Shit. I've seen enough paranormal videos to know this is bad, or potentially a good sign for me.

I am not the only one here.

The loss of power means I am not alone.

Hello? I squeak.

I always laugh at these moments on YouTube; people enter these churches, old asylums, and abandoned hospitals, primed and ready to come face-to-mist with a paranormal entity, but when it actually happens, they freak the fuck out and start losing their shit. In some countries, praying to a god or gods seems to help, while in other locations, screaming curse words and kicking whatever is closest seems to ward off the evil spirits (and make for excellent viewing).

Now here I am in my abandoned tunnel, wanting to meet something from the other side while simultaneously losing my cool. I've noticed Americans don't have a standard *we pray or we curse and kick shit* response. It's basically run, meet the ghost head-on, or find a corner to scream and cry in, Blair Witch style.

I stand there and wait. I want to see this entity, this thing, this wisp/fog/whatever it is. I don't think anything will actually materialize in front of me, but I don't want to be the person who runs.

I never have been.

I didn't run from my brain surgery.

I didn't run from my chemo or radiation.

I didn't flee from my friends when they ran from me.

I flick the button on my headlamp, but nothing happens. I just charged the device, so I know it should be working. The spirit box won't turn on, so I'm by myself here.

And then I see her.

I feel her.

Every part of my right side, my bad side freezes, which means something is definitely happening. Goosebumps rise on the left half of my body—a weird quirk of surgery, I don't get them on my right side any longer. I feel like I might pass out, so although I'm still seated, I steady myself on the stone of #17.

This is what you wanted. I'm not sure if I'm hearing this aloud, or it's just what's left of my brain.

Not quite a figure, the foggy entity floats by gently and without concern for me or my malfunctioning equipment. This isn't the tunnel with the bride who lost her betrothed, or the tunnel with the horrible wreck. It's just a bypassed tunnel on the Rail Trail where some shit happened on some day that no one probably remembers, which makes this incident far more fascinating to me.

Who was this ghost? Was it a spirit at all or just some left-over energy from stuff that happened long ago?

I believe this is an interactive, intelligent being; more than residual energy, this spirit has something to say to me, something to impart, something important to tell me.

I need to listen, and I don't need paranormal equipment for this. I need to sit and hear the shadows, to hear what the wind needs to say. I can't run from this, and I can't pretend I don't know what's going on.

I lean back in the lantern alcove and rest my senses. These places are the only landmarks where I get any peace. When I reopen my eyes, the foggy figure stands still a few feet from me, and if she had eyes, I swear she would be looking back.

Of course, she can't speak, but I swear she does.

I stick out my hand and feel the coldness of a hallway with a window left open late at night.

The spirit and I are one in this moment, and I don't feel lonely—I feel heard and understood. We float in this tunnel together, and no one can tell me otherwise. We belong here. I don't need to know her name or what happened to her, though I feel like it might predate this structure. She's young, but between me and the age of the bride in Tunnel #19. She's here in this space to protect people like me.

You don't belong here yet. Not all the time. You're just visiting.

Water in the tunnel drips. My headlamp flickers like an old candle.

It's time for me to leave, but I don't want to.

I want to sit here forever with my hand in her nebulous stomach until she tells me I have to go because I'm not done living yet.

Harrisville, West Virginia

I decide to give Tinder one last shot.

I upload a single picture: It's the headshot I use for my faculty page at Appalachian State. It's not edited, there's no filter, and it's unequivocally me.

I use the initial Z.

No, it's not my actual initial, but I'm pissed off by the

behavior of every man I've been in contact with throughout the past year, and I'm doing things my way now, so I pick a distinctive letter from the middle of my first name.

The bio sections?

Completely blank.

I swipe a few times before I come across a blurry pic of a guy named Jeramy. He has a skull cap and a beard, but I can see a kindness in his eyes, even from the distance.

Sure, why not?

I swipe right. A few minutes later, he strikes up a conversation. I'm bored enough to entertain it. To my surprise, he asks me out for coffee within a few lines.

What?

This is unprecedented.

I've entertained months of texting from multiple men now, and so far, I've done the heavy lifting.

Sure, I respond, though I'm not actually *that* sure I want to do this. He lives in Athens, Ohio, so we decide to meet in Parkersburg, which is about halfway for both of us. I recommend the coffee shop Stoked, and he agrees.

Then I panic.

Wait, I type, *what's your Covid protocol been?*

I usually ask this right away, but he threw me off by suggesting a date so quickly. Usually, men play the pen pal game for at least a couple of months, and I can figure out just how safe sexually (if I want) and Covidly (because I must) they have been.

I had it in September pretty bad, he responds, and I breathe.[2]

Jeramy had survived.

Oh, I'm so sorry! I respond, though I am also relieved and excited to meet him. I turned away from a lot of prospects when I discovered they didn't take Covid protocols seriously.

It's okay. It sucked but I got through it.

That must have been tough.

To be honest, it's nice to discuss someone else's medical struggles for once. I also slow myself down a bit with the texting. I usually start blowing up anyone who shows a modicum of interest, but a new Suzanne lives on Tinder now.

Shit.

It's okay.

My name is Suzanne, by the way. I got tired of people knowing too much about me on here.

Yeah, lot of creeps. I understand.

There's no way he could understand.

Although I said I would wait a bit longer this time, I give Jeramy my actual cell phone number. He seems genuinely nice, and texting through the app is as annoying as all the catfishing and ghosting. Once Jeramy has my number, I still keep the texts short and avoid the urge to spew out paragraph after paragraph of my thoughts and opinions and questions about his life.

It's finally occurred to me that perhaps I might scare some people.

I'd like to see another picture of you? he texts.

Okay.

Here we go.

If you've been on Tinder as a straight or bi female for more than seven seconds, you know most men just want naked pictures. When porn anyone and everyone can see is no longer enough, they need to feel special and want *individual shots* they think no one else gets.

I send Jeramy another picture of my smiling face.

What I don't realize at the time is that 90 days earlier, Jeramy went on a date with a woman from Huntington he met on Tinder. She **kittenfished (v.)** him, or **showed up to the date looking quite different than her pictures,**

heavier and nothing like he'd seen before because she couldn't use filters in real life. Jeramy, as always, was a gentleman and bought her lunch, said it was nice to meet her, walked her to her car, and wished her well. Because he didn't give her the hookup she desired, he got home to discover he'd been reported by her to Tinder and had a 90-day ban.

He never knew what she reported him for—it could have been anything, but they were all lies—but I apparently swiped right on his first day back.

If she hadn't reported him, we would have likely never met, so thank you, random girl, for your kittenfishing.

Your gorgeous, Jeramy responds to my picture.

Ahhh. The your/you're mistake makes me twitch. However, I let it go. I am not going to push someone away, someone who seems extremely nice, based on a grammatical error.

I have seen what else is out there.[3]

Thank you!

I'll stop blowing you up now, he responds.

I don't mind, I say, but he doesn't know how I'm refusing to text a bunch before meeting up. It's better this way, I convince myself.

Don't let them in too easily.

Maintain the mystery as long as I can.

New Milton, West Virginia, Sherwood Tunnel, #4, 846 ft.

My parents think I have lost my mind.

I am constantly bored and searching for a larger purpose.

And that's how I end up in New Milton, WV, on a 65-degree day in October when it was actually supposed to snow.

Welcome to West Virginia.

The Sherwood Tunnel sounds like it should be in the 12th or 13th century, hiding Robinhood in the honeysuckle decorating its stone. I'm impressed the tunnel actually has a brightness the others do not. The Sherwood Tunnel features English ivy hanging from the entrance in willowy wisps and other inviting greenery hugging the stone, almost as if the other side will open up to a vivid forest for those who dare to pass through the dauting darkness.

I am slightly disappointed there is only a trail on the other side, but I remind myself I knew this all along.

Sometimes my imagination gets away from me.

Harrisville, West Virginia

I am silently crying on the bathroom floor again.

The shower.

Over the sink.

I have cried here so many times since moving home, for myriad reasons.

The cancer. (Is it back? Did it ever really leave? Malignant brain cancers always leave cells behind, so sometimes they just hang out there and wait.) No one but Kate and my other coworkers believing CK pushed me into a wall. *We just don't want to talk about it.* Oh, I'm sorry you don't want to talk about how someone we both know abused me, but it happened, and it can't unhappen, and nothing anyone says will change it. Somehow that makes it my fault for talking about it after she blew it up all over Boone anyway. Dave stonewalling me after screaming at me at 6 a.m. each morning. That hot water mixed with tears sure made me feel like I was at the ocean, everyone! All the Tinder boys who led me on. All the Tinder boys I let lead me on because I had trouble drawing boundaries.

And now I'm crying because I'm just over it all.

How will this date I'm supposed to go on today be different?

He will probably just be another dick who isn't really interested or drops me as soon as I let loose The Abridged Version of *Frontal Matter* on him, which, if I do go on this date, I plan to do before the night ends.

It's only fair.

I'm supposed to go on a date today. I don't want to, I text Timmathew. As much as I hate to admit it, Timmathew is one of my only friends. Besides Emily, who is probably tired of hearing me whine about my bad luck in love, Timmathew responds to my texts when no one else does. Sure, he catfished and breadcrumbed me like a motherfucker, but I don't care about that anymore. I need a friend, and I think he can handle this.

Maybe I just needed a friend all along.

Sure, he's an asshole, but so am I, I guess.

You should go! He responds. *You never know what might happen.*

For once, I decide Timmathew could be right. If I'm going to go, I need to go now. I don't have time for a shower or multiple outfit changes, so I throw on some mascara and tell my parents I'm meeting an old friend in Parkersburg.

You're going to Parkiesburg tonight? my dad asks.

He doesn't actually call the town Parkiesburg.

No, tomorrow night. That's why I'm busy getting ready.

She's not a teenager anymore, Ted, my mom says.

Well, then she can stop backtalking me like one.

I need to get out of this house.

We may agree on nothing, but I do appreciate the freedom my mom gives me, despite living under their roof.

It's going to be dark out, my dad says.

Yes, it gets dark at 4 p.m. now, but that doesn't mean I'm going to shut myself in a casket and call it a night.

Without me realizing it, the season has shifted to fall.

I don't wait for anyone to answer; this guy said he's bringing pumpkin bread, so if he sucks, at least I can bring home some snacks. My parents aren't known for keeping food in the house.

I am not stoked about going to Stoked, but I'm going to make it work.

Forty-five minutes later, I nearly run over Jeramy.

He looks panicked as he runs to his car, and I wonder if he's trying to bounce before I show up.

Turns out he forgot the pumpkin bread, but I forgive him.

Much to my ultimate surprise, I instantaneously feel comfortable with Jeramy.

You look like you're from Boone, I tell him, because he does. He has a full light brown beard, soulful blue eyes, and manly hands.

You're actually not the first person to tell me that.

He needs to be chopping wood somewhere.

The Stoked dining area isn't open because of Covid, so we use the drive-through and try to sit outside; unfortunately, I keep shivering, so we spend the majority of our first date in his car, which reeks of cigarette smoke. Instead of being grossed out, I feel at home. My sister's cars[4] always smell like a tobacco store.

Although I don't realize this at the time, Jeramy isn't much of a talker.

Despite this, we fall into a conversational rhythm like an old folk song. I don't feel nervous. For the first time in a long time, I feel like I can breathe normally without crashing waves of crippling anxiety. I don't feel the need to divulge my big *brain cancer secret.* We discuss everything from his time with Covid to me almost accidentally smashing him with my car.

As we get to know each other, I forget about my infinite loneliness and *disorganized attachment style.*

I don't analyze anything.

I forget about Timmatthew. I forget about Josh. I forget about Marcus flashing me and everyone else in the Ohio park last summer. I forget about the patterns of abuse I keep falling into, and the way I keep letting people treat me because I think I don't deserve more.

I just have a nice, normal time.

Are you hungry? Jeramy asks.

I am.

We drive around for a good twenty minutes, searching for an open restaurant. Finally, we find a Mexican spot where we are the only two patrons abiding by the mask mandate. I try to hide my disappointment when my plate arrives with a giant pile of tomatoes.

I might vomit, though.

Nothing, not even chemo, makes me want to vomit more than tomatoes.

Are you okay? Jeramy asks.

Fuck. I've never been good at hiding my feelings, and apparently, this guy can already read me.

Swell.

I'm great! I really am great. I'm having a good time, the best time, truly, and I'm not going to let a pile of chopped tomatoes ruin this, dammit. I notice Jeramy has already finished his plate.

I didn't even see what was on it.

The meal ends faster than I anticipated, and when we step outside, a magical thin layer of snow has coated the ground, and I feel like we are in a movie. I can't believe I almost didn't show up, pumpkin bread or not.

Jeramy apparently doesn't want the night to end either, so we drive back to Stoked and sit in his car a bit longer. We see an animal that looks like a wolf sniffing the sugary snow; we allow our imaginations to take us to the fantastical before we realize it's actually just a big Husky, but we have fun with the image.

I feel comfortable enough to discuss *everything that happened* and hope he doesn't run away. My logic is as follows: If he does want to take off, it's the end of the night, so at least it was a good date. If he doesn't want to follow up, at least he wasn't a creep. We both had a good time.

He seems to take it well.

I end the night by asking if I can give him a hug.

It's a bit awkward, but somehow, we are both to blame.

By the time I get home, I have a text.

Hope you got home okay. Had a good time tonight!

I smile.

Things should always be this easy.

Dallison, West Virginia, Eaton/Bee Tree Tunnel, #21, 2030 ft.

I am familiar with Dallison, West Virginia; my mom drove my sister and I here on Sunday afternoons without fail for baton lessons with the Roth family, wonderful people who taught me to love the art and sport of baton twirling. Close to *Parkiesburg* but still very much rural West Virginia, the trail is as deserted.

Empty.

Eerie, even.

Apparently, this was once an actual town called Eaton, and I can't imagine anyone living here.

I don't even hear any animals.

The entire time I walk, I feel as if I'm being watched—not by woodland creatures but by something or someone I'll never see.

When I reach the tunnel after about three miles, I get an even more troubled feeling than I had on the trail. This entire area has an aura of malaise I can't shake; I don't even want to enter this tunnel, which is odd. I've never felt scared to go into any of them.

I'm a bit surprised because as creepy and bizarre as all of these tunnels are, the current Bee Tree/Eaton Tunnel has been rebuilt since the strangest event occurred.

According to old newspapers and Mr. Samples, who has an uncanny memory for dates and historical tragedies, in 1963, workers were performing repairs on tunnels when quite suddenly, everything collapsed. No one knew who or what to blame, and quite honestly, it was a bit early for The Mothman. The stone from the tunnel caved in and crashed around the workers; while some escaped the rubble, rocks crushed the more unfortunate. Although West Virginians were not strangers to collapsing structures, they most often happened in coal mines. With three men trapped inside the tunnel, no one knew what to do.

Rescuers saved one man.

A broken ankle.

They then saved another.

He later died due to his injuries.

A third man never made it out, and the original Eaton/Bee Tree Tunnel, now collapsed and caved in directly above the newer structure, now serves as the man's tragic burial site.

But first, I must traverse the new tunnel, which is a graffi-tied mess.

It's midday but feels more like dusk. I don't want to walk through this tunnel, but the quest called and I answered. My stomach drops as I enter the archway, and I remind myself: No one actually died here.

This is the new one.

The Eaton/Bee Tree Tunnel has more graffiti than the other sites I've visited, perhaps because it's closer to the city. West Virginia doesn't really have urban areas, not comparatively, but this one is closer to civilization than the others on the more rural trails. I can imagine kids cutting school early and bumming around here with spray paint, pretending they are in gangs that don't actually exist. (Perhaps in the areas of WV near D.C., Pittsburgh, Charleston, and Huntington there might be gangs, but anything near here would be nothing more than a group of teenagers bored with the playground.)

Still, I am nervous there might be a person in this tunnel, a real, live person, not a trapped spirit, who might try to harm me. I have pepper spray, but with my phone and water bottle, I don't know how easily and quickly I could get to it if I needed to.

The persistent quiet unnerves me.

I cannot run. I don't think I'll ever be able to run. Sure, I can walk faster now, but running is not an option.

I am not worried about this tunnel caving in, but everything seems heavy.

I feel watched.

FUCK EVERYONE.

MICHAEL LOVES MARIA SO STAY AWAY JOHN YOU BASTARD.

GODDAMNFUCKITYFUCK-FUCKSCREWSCHOOL.

Maybe I shouldn't be scared. This just seems like a bunch of harmless graffiti, but someone could so easily be hiding in one of these lantern crevasses, ready to jump out and strangle me.

I don't think I took a breath the entire time I walked through the tunnel.

The name through me off a bit—when I heard Bee Tree

Tunnel, I was expecting something cute, like something you might see painted in a child's bedroom.

But now.

I must find the collapsed tunnel.

I don't see anything.

I know from my tunnel hunting experience (most people in these parts hunt deer; I hunt tunnels), they are sneaky structures and especially if they have been bypassed, or overtaken by trees, grass, and other natural elements. However, as I look around the area, I see absolutely nothing and wonder if I missed it on the other side.

Then I glance at a small footpath up a hillside.

This has to be it, but I don't see anything up there.

I expect to view a bunch of rubble, but there's nothing.

I need to venture upward.

This isn't safe.

I don't care.

I have to crawl up a perilously muddy, rocky path to see this original collapsed tunnel-graveyard, but I'm not missing this opportunity.

I just hope it's actually up there.

I leave my water bottle below and find a sturdy stick to help me out. At least I brought gloves. Instead of shielding me from the cold, they will assist me in my climb.

There isn't much left of the collapsed tunnel: some old mossed over rocks and a brass switch key to commemorate the dead. I don't know if the key is in memoriam or an original.

I sit up there for quite some time, thinking about what's to come.

Harrisville, West Virginia

I have one non-tunnel related item on my bucket list to complete: start a literary journal.

I don't think I will be able to do this.

I want to so badly, but with my memory issues and stretches to keep myself employed, this is all too daunting.

I casually mention this to Emily, and she says, *You know what? We should start one. There are 18-year-olds on Twitter doing it. There's no reason we can't.*

I am intrigued.

I do not have an active Twitter account.

Pause

Emily and I have had innumerable creative projects since we were small children. We inflamed our parents' ears with songs we wrote and recorded on tape decks when we were ten. We were early podcast innovators as we sat for hours and recorded ourselves talking about whatever preteen girls felt like discussing in the early 90s. As teenagers, we decided to write something called *the alt.novel*, which was some version of hybrid writing about a band that didn't exist. Not surprisingly, the alt.novel never made it to the presses as a book or a concept.

End Pause

We call the journal *Dead Skunk Mag* as a homage to a song our fathers' band, The Samples Brothers, repurposed many nights for folky crowds of flat foot dancing fans across Appalachia.

To our surprise, the literary magazine takes off.

People actually want to be a part of it.

We both start finding a larger purpose in showcasing the creative writing of others. We become the first publication for a young woman majoring in creative writing, and she thanks us profusely. The story, which we suspect to be thinly-veiled fiction about choosing a university, details her experience connecting with her father when visiting schools. Her school, known for creative writing, tags Dead Skunk in a social media post.

Emily and I beam with pride.

This feels good.

I start finding gems and *taking on projects* requiring me to work closely with writers to whittle giant fiction pieces into three-paragraph flash stories.

I love this.

Sometimes I pretend I don't, but I do.

Sometimes really weird shit happens, like Emily receiving poems about *fucking Jesus* or writers sending really strange bio information we didn't ask for or need.

Sometimes we take the good with the bad.

I don't know what will happen when I'm gone, but I hope Emily always stays slightly left of center.

Walker, West Virginia, Rodimer's Tunnel, Tunnel #22, 338 ft.

After finding The Eaton Tunnel, I decide to make it a Double Tunnel Day.

In other words, I want to hide from my family.

I'll bring them home Olive Garden to make up for it. I actually go to Outback and get a cheeseburger for my dad, but he always remarks, *Suzanne, Olive Garden makes the best burgers.*

My mom and I laugh.

Rodimer's Tunnel isn't far from The Eaton Tunnel, so I keep hiking. It's drizzling, but it's always like this in West Virginia.

My right-side weakness creeps up on me after the long Eaton hike, but I take my chances. The area stays still, quiet, and creepy and once I find Rodimer's Tunnel, the inkling only increases.

I feel like I don't belong, and dammit, the hills have eyes.

Though Rodimer's Tunnel doesn't have the lore of the Eaton Tunnel, the east portal is completely caved in and destroyed.

I get the fucking West Virginia willies.

I still step into the tunnel, as is my custom, but then I urgently turn around and begin the walk back to the car.

If I could run, I would.

Harrisville, West Virginia

I don't have a karaoke song, but if I did, it would be "Heartbeat City" by The Cars.

Everyone would be bored as fuck except my dad.

He introduced me to The Cars, and with the barn door separating our living quarters, we turn the song on full blast when my mom leaves the house.

Moonville, Ohio

Jeramy says he has somewhere special to take me, and I have no idea where we are going. We have been *seeing each other* for a while now, and it's actually going well.

Though it's not far from my home, I'm not familiar with the Athens area. I can't tell from Jeramy's face where we might be headed. After a short drive, he parks at a trailhead; I am excited for a nice hike he has planned. I'm assuming he has scoped this place out and made certain it's nice and flat. It's a sunny day, so I'm excited to be outside.

I am surprised to see how many people are out on the trail. I am spoiled by North Bend during the weekdays when myself and sometimes a birdwatcher are the only wanderers on the old tracks.

We walk for a bit, and I have some issues. It's not quite as flat as I hoped, and I'm a bit disappointed Jeramy hasn't picked up on what I can and can't do yet. I have to grab his arm to stay afloat in the sea of sticks, mud, rocks, and people. Without him, I would not be able to navigate this trail.

Jeramy gives me a guided tour of a ghost town as we walk. *This was the community known as Moonville. It was an actual place in the 1900s, and now it's a ghost town. Up until a few years ago, you could actually find remnants of Moonville, but people have looted everything at this point.* We are deep in the woods, and it seems impossible this could have been an actual thriving place at any point. It didn't succeed for that long, I guess. *Eventually, the train had to stop going through here because it just wasn't worth it.* He dramatically pauses. *Yellow fever, starvation. Legend has it Moonville citizens would just grab provisions—or even people—off the cars, but the conductors just refused to stop. It was too dangerous. Some of the people they grabbed just ended up living in Moonville until the bitter end.*

He's a fantastic storyteller, and I think he knows. Soft spoken but confident, you can actually hear a fire crackling around his voice when he tells stories like this.

Until the bitter end?

There's a Moonville Cemetery for the ones who didn't make it...which was everyone. It was the early 1900s, and this is Southern Ohio. People didn't have cars or transportation or the means to leave. Especially the ones who got ripped off the train. If they didn't die from impact, they starved. Without resources, everyone starved to death anyway.[5]

I'd like to say I'm horrified, but I'm more intrigued than anything.

It takes me a minute to realize—we are on an old train track.

Then I see a tunnel.

A TUNNEL! I yell.

You didn't expect that? Come on.

But I really didn't. I was so caught up in navigating the terrain and then the fantastic campfire story, I wasn't thinking about a tunnel.

I am thrilled as I see the stone archway ahead. The Moonville Tunnel[6] looks like every other one I've seen so far, but it's the thought that counts.

Finally, someone gets me.

* * *

I am jazzed on the way back to Jeramy's house. The day could not have gone better. Sure, we haven't officially said we are dating or anything yet, but do we need to? We both said we deleted Tinder after I went to his house the first time and met his cat, the gorgeous Wild Kitty, with her giant green eyes and deviant Maine Coon fur.

I spent the night, we kissed, and it felt right.

It was good. Really good, he said. I don't feel pressure to define things any further. We've been doing this a few months, and it is falling into place, like the stones on the still-standing Moonville Tunnel. I will ride this proverbial train to Moonville until I fall off and starve, I guess.

I want to talk to you about something, Jeramy says as we step back into his house. He hands me a Coke, which I'm not really supposed to have because of my diabetes, but I've been drinking them when I visit him on the weekends. We call these Big Coke Parties, although the drinks are normal sized.

Dammit. This doesn't sound good. I can feel the tension, and it feels like one of the Moonville ghosts followed us home.

I'm moving to a place called Pullman, Washington, this summer, Jeramy says. *Greek House Chefs is promoting me.*[7]

Fuck.

Of course.

I finally find someone I really like, someone who treats me well, someone I actually get along with and the dynamic between us isn't toxic, and he's moving across the country.

I know how this goes. He's about to say *this has been really fun, I've enjoyed getting to know you, you're a really cool girl, I'd love to hang out with you before I leave, but if you're not okay with that, I understand.*

Oh, I say and take a swig of Coke.

And I'd like for you to come with me.

I taste the Coke in my mouth and focus on the feeling of the sugar rotting my teeth. Is he really asking me to move across the country with him after dating a few months? I look at his pale blue eyes, waiting for me to answer. I know I could answer him now or later, and he wouldn't mind.

I want to answer him now because I know.

I'd love to, I say.

I've always been a bit impulsive, but I know this is right. I want to do this with Jeramy. He surprised me with a tunnel, accepted me with brain cancer and all, and cares for me better than anyone ever has.

For the first time in a long time, I feel safe with someone.

Granted the bar was low, but I truly feel safe.

Safe.

I can't overestimate the significance of that word.

When do we leave?

Salem-ish Area, West Virginia, Brandy Gap Tunnel, #2, 1086 ft. & Trough Tunnel #3, caved in

I cannot find the final two tunnels.

Like glioblastoma cells, they seem impossible to pin down.

I've tried different GPS locations, driving, walking, and a combination of both. No tunnels and not even a trail in sight. I might be crazy. They might not exist at all and could be some strange figment of my brain cancer has caused. Thirteen tunnels on the North Bend Rail Trail? Sure thing, Suzanne. Whatever you say.

I don't want to ask for help, but I don't know what else to do.

Jeramy and I are getting ready to move thousands of miles away, and I need to find these last two tunnels to complete my quest.

He visits me at my parents' house on a Saturday, and we end up on a dirt road in Doddridge County. Jeramy says, *I'm sorry, sugar, but I don't think we're going to be able to find them. My car isn't going to make it down these roads.* I tell him I understand and try to hold back tears.

I cry way too much.

I get quiet; Jeramy knows how upset I am, how much this meant to me.

It meant everything.

I have an idea, he says.

He whips his car around and somehow finds the main road again. I don't know how he does it, but he finds a trailhead.

One problem: According to Jeramy's driving calculations, the tunnels are close together but about six miles down the trailhead, and it's raining. Neither of us want to do this walk, but Jeramy thinks we can easily find the tunnels now.

We locate the trail.

We look at the sign on the trailhead that clearly states ONLY AUTHORIZED VEHICLES.

Clearly, non-authorized vehicles have been on this trail; it's Doddridge County.

It's a rainy Tuesday afternoon.

Jeramy guns it down the rocks and dirt.

We stop right outside of the Brandy Gap Tunnel. I am amazed to finally be here. After everything I've been through, I'm so close to completing my tunnel quest I don't care if it's raining or how we got here. Although I originally wanted to complete the search for the tunnels alone, it feels right for Jeramy to be with me.

Brandy Gap feels haunted. I had read there was a cemetery nearby, but Jeramy and I have other pursuits to follow. Brandy Gap may be haunted as fuck, but I set out to find the thirteen tunnels, and we are losing daylight.

I don't have time for cemeteries today.

Enough time for that in the future.

We creep through the Brandy Gap Tunnel and make shadow puppets with our headlamps like little kids. It's safer in here than it is outside in the rain. As we are about to leave, we see a shadow figure neither of us made at the other end of the tunnel.

Did you see that? he asks. *What the fuck is that smell?*

What the hell? I say, and it echoes because I am loud.

I spot a black, shadowy feminine figure floating out of the Brandy Gap Tunnel exit, and I am frozen in place. I think I've got to be seeing things, but Jeramy saw her as well. She looked nothing like a ghost but instead had pronged fork-like fingers, a hoop skirt, three discs for a waist, Mothman-red eyes, and a head shaped like a Maple leaf.[8]

You know I'm just messing with you, right? Jeramy says, but I'm not too sure.

Something was there something was there something was there.

* * *

217

There's bad news about Tunnel #3.

Just as I couldn't find it anywhere on a map, neither can Jeramy. It was bypassed by the trail, that much I know, but past that, we don't have any information. However, we have a car nearby, and we know it's not behind us. When we hit the trailhead, nothing was in the rearview but dilapidated houses and chained-up dogs, so the tunnel has to be in front of us.

Please? I beg. *I really need to do this.*

I can tell Jeramy would rather get in the car and go home, but he indulges me. Some women need diamonds or promises of marriages, but I just want a chance to see this tunnel.

As someone who often forages for mushrooms and other fun woodland items, he spots the tunnel before I do. Number Three is, by far, the most crumbled, ruined tunnel of them all. Bypassed by the trail, the tunnel has fallen in on itself like an abandoned building left to rot and decay.

I don't really think you should go in that one, Jeramy says.

I don't disagree with him, but I do want to step inside a little bit. I have to: It's a requirement of my search.

I flip on the headlamp and take a peek in the tunnel. It's an odd feeling, this one. I can't quite place it.

It feels like something bad happened here, Jeramy says, and I remember my fifth-grade year. We were moving within the county, and my parents found a deal on a gorgeous two-story house they wanted to check out.

I stepped inside and said, *Someone died in here.*

Oh hush, my mom yell-whispered as she poked me in the shoulder as the real estate agent bucked her teeth at me. *They did not. Stop that.*

I was a well-mannered child but not always able to keep my mouth shut, especially if I thought places, we might end up living were haunted. The house had plush green carpeting and meticulous matching ivy wallpaper (wallpaper was still very much fashionable in early 1990s WV décor), and I'm sure my mom couldn't believe the deal she and my dad might get on this funeral home.

As we paraded around, the feeling inside me grew heavier and heavier, like a black balloon being filled with helium inside my stomach. We *could not* live here. Something horrible had happened in this house, and no amount of green carpet and matching ivy wallpaper could ever cover it up.

I would have none of it.

We ended up putting a doublewide by my grandparents' house and living there happilyeverafter until 2021, and a few months after settling into our cedar doublewide (that looked very much like a regular house), my mom sat me down at the table and said, *I'm going to tell you this once and then walk away. Someone did die in that house we looked at. That's all I'm going to say.* Then, just as she said she would, she stood up, walked away in her Princess Diana style, and I asked zero questions about it.

That's a long-winded side story to say this tunnel feels exactly the same way.

I have zero info on this tunnel, except that it was bypassed and caved in.

There's water dripping, but there's always water dripping in these things.

This time, the bad feeling is mostly Jeramy's.

I just feel like something really weird happened here, he says, *like maybe a sexual assault.*

I don't doubt him.

The tunnels are full of residual energy.

I hope to leave some good behind.

We pause for a moment to take a picture. Jeramy hates pictures, but I want to remember this, and he obliges. The rain actually quits for a moment, and a glint of sun shows the tunnel behind us, bad energy and all.

I want my smile to leave some good behind.

And then the rain comes again, hard. I can't run, but we pull up our hoods and walk as quickly as we can back to his car. Near the trail, we hear a not-so-friendly dog growling and howling. People live near these trails and sometimes, it's easy to miss the houses alongside the pathways. We can only hope the dog is sequestered in the yard or porch.

Then we hear the gunshot.

What the hell?

We don't know where the gunshot came from, where it was aimed, or who shot it, but we finally make it back to the car alive. Jeramy tears back down the trail illegally but without bullet holes in the tires or car doors.

I have done it.

Thirteen tunnels.

PART IV
ON THE MOVE

Harrisville, West Virginia

In my final farewell to the Country Roads, The Midnight Cowboy helps Jeramy pack up the Penske so we can make our way to Washington.

I have more animals than possessions.

Well, maybe books, though I did try to give some to our sweet neighbor.

The Midnight Cowboy wants to make conversation, manly conversation with Jeramy and my dad, but we need to get on the road. Assuming we don't have any disasters, the trip will take a little past a week, and with The Midnight Cowboy telling Jeramy stories about Harrisville in 1993, maybe longer.

Also, there seems to be some confusion about what goes in the Penske, and my mom has to keep going out to get what belongs to her and toting it back into their house with a worried expression on her face that I might *steal the Shark Vacuum.*

Princess Peppermint seems to understand we are all leaving and looks pissed about the noise but relieved her nemesis, Delilah, will be gone forever. She stares at us with her menacing blue eyes and subtly growls when anyone steps too close to her rug or her food. I can see in her face how she plans to take over *my apartment* the minute I'm gone. Although I tried to be her friend, she only sees me as The Enemy Who Brought Other Animals into My Fortress.

So long, Princess Peppermint. Thanks for all the hisses and growls, girlfriend.

I will miss her.

My parents and I act like we won't miss each other.

We've never been especially affectionate.

As I leave West Virginia, I think about healing. How I arrived broken and am leaving with a renewed source of life. How I walked through thirteen dark tunnels and somehow came out on the other side alive.

Greenville, Ohio

Our first stop is Greenville, Ohio: Jeramy's hometown. The Penske's been swerving all over the road like a drunk driver, but we attribute this to all the shit in the back. My car, stuffed with live animals, does just fine.

So far, no one, including myself, has pissed or shit in the vehicle.

If anyone does, we might have to throw the whole thing away.

Jeramy's told me his mom's husband (she remarried long after Jeramy was an adult, so it feels wrong to say *stepdad*) is a farmer, so I'm expecting a West Virginia farm in the state next door.

What I'm not expecting is the type of farm people spend years making in those simulation games, replete with a giant trucking fleet and an entire apartment, probably the size of the apartment I left in Boone, just for the farmers to use during the day.

Jeramy really undersold this whole *my mom is married to a farmer thing.*

His mom is married to a businessman who happens to know how to farm.

I can't hide my surprise as I see the fleet of trucks and acres upon acres of crops. The house is, of course, nice, and I forget what houses look like when you *aren't pet people.* You don't have to mask any weird smells or constantly scrape fur or puke off carpet.

His mom and stepdad are wonderful. I meet Jeramy's Papaw, a gruff fellow who was a butcher, loves the Cincinnati Reds, and hotdogs, and we connect immediately over a game of marbles. I like him as much as I like the fresh fish on the grill, and Jeramy seems surprised. To this day, the first question Pap asks Jeramy on the phone is, *How's your friend?* and I beam brighter than a headlamp in a dark tunnel.

But something is bothering me.

Before we left Athens, Jeramy told me about spending time with his old friend Courtney. *She said you must be cool because you didn't mind us hanging out together.* I didn't mind them hanging out together at all, but Jeramy told me her fiancé was coming with her.

Wait, I said in the Penske parking lot. *I thought her fiancé was coming too.*

Well, he was but he couldn't.

He won't look me in the eye.

I don't care at all he spent time with a female friend, but I do care if he lied to me. Sitting at his mom's house on her porch and looking out at the wind turbines on fields that last forever, I ask him one more time.

Was Courtney's fiancé ever coming to hang out?

I don't know why it's that big of a deal. Why are you jealous of her?

I'm not jealous at all. I was hanging out with Travis that day, so it would be quite a double standard if I was hanging out with a guy friend and jealous of your female friend. It just... doesn't sound like something a girl would say if her fiancé was ever going to be there.

Okay, fine. I lied. You just seem like a jealous girlfriend, so I figured I'd be better off lying.

I'm about to lose it. Here I am moving across the country with a liar who thinks I'm jealous, and it's too late to back out now.

What made you think that? I ask.

That one time you sent me a text that said, "Did you take a survey?" when I said people were acting weird because of a full moon.

You've got to be kidding me. I remember the text, and it was pure sarcasm and not related to jealousy at all. Instead of asking if I was actually jealous, he just assumed I was, and now it's led to this.

Lying.

Deceit.

Moving across the country with someone I don't know if I can trust.

Really? You've got to be kidding me.

It's just a white lie.

A white lie is when you say, "I ate toast for breakfast" when you actually ate oatmeal. Don't give me that shit.

But we must keep moving, white lies or even darker truths.

Jeramy's family is wonderful and kind, and I don't want to leave.

.   .   .

Waterloo, Iowa

Twenty minutes outside Waterloo, we hit roadwork.

No big deal. We have had a decent trip so far with very little hassle. All pets remain alive and hydrated, I haven't had any speeding tickets yet, and I'm a third of the way through *Infinite Jest*, though I'm not even sure I want to finish it.

Then it happens.

Perhaps the cancer won't kill me.

I see Jeramy swerve with the Penske before I see the giant piece of plastic blocking the road. As someone who grew up in West Virginia, I'm well aware *Watch for deer!* means *I love you!*, but I've never had the chance to practice my MarioKart skills quite like this before. I somehow cleanly escape the enormous plastic chunk, and everything seems fantastic, though I don't understand why no one working on the interstate has tried to move the obstacle yet.

Anyway.

Ten minutes outside Waterloo.

We just need to get through this remaining roadwork.

Suddenly, the sky rains rubber.

The rubber rain nearly shatters the windshield of the tiny Scion. I have to keep driving because if I don't, I will crash myself and the mini zoo into the Midwestern roadside attractions of construction cutouts and traffic cones.

Jeramy has no idea.

I frantically call him, and we pull off the interstate.

The cats wail like baby cougars abandoned in the wild. My car says it's 93 degrees outside.

Gatsby pants.

The right back tire on the car tow of the Penske is completely blown.

Motherfucker.

We were so close to our hotel.

I follow the Brokse off the road and park behind the collapsed moving truck. Jeramy is sweaty and tired. I am afraid of someone swerving off the road and mangling me. Wild Kitty, Jeramy's cat, looks ready to run back to her feral beginnings in the woods. He tells me to head to the hotel, get some food, and go to bed.

I hope I don't look as relieved as I feel.

I also feel awful that Jeramy has to wait in the Iowa sun, which is more vicious than one might imagine, for an unnamed number of hours for the Brokse repair people. I find the hotel easily but stop at a gas station first.

Waterloo, Iowa, has more face tattoos and motorbikes than anywhere I've ever been before.

I pick up some iced tea and Jack Daniels at the gas station.

I don't know who will need it more, me or Jeramy, but I feel it's my duty to indulge in this overpriced gas station whiskey. Is it overpriced because it's in a gas station or because we are getting further from Tennessee? I don't have time to wonder; I have three angry cats and a confused geriatric dog in the car.

I'm also almost out of gas, as one always is with a miniature vehicle, and I need to fill up because I don't think I will make it across the street to the hotel.

And people in Waterloo, Iowa, are hostile as fuck.

Something about all the cement, sun, and tattoo ink must have done something to their psyches.

THIS ALL FOR YOU?

Yes.

K.

He does not offer me a bag. Everywhere else I've lived has this bizarre rule where you have to carry all alcohol out of stores in a bag to preserve Southern and Appalachian appearances, I suppose.

Welcome to the central Midwest, baby.

A motorbikist with a spider tattoo crawling up his face nearly runs me over.

I don't wanna die in Waterloo.

* * *

The hotel clerk is new and, if I had to guess, on meth.

Okay so I literally like have you checked into room 114 Beth that's like the one oh my god I can't feel my face right now I need to clean this desk or something that's the one three down from the outside door and yeah that's totally like literally fine you have cats and a dog and like we literally don't care about that at all I like love to clean so much so here's your key.

My boyfriend is coming later tonight in a Penske with a car tow. Where should he park it?

The hotel clerk has danced, shimmied really, to the bottom of the desk where I can't see her. I get a glimpse of a neck flower tat when she grows her way back up to me.

Oh, like literally anywhere is freaking fine! We like don't care.

What I didn't think about was getting the cats into the hotel room. Though I've been getting stronger and feeling better lately, two of our three precious kittens weigh over twenty pounds. *Mostly fur!* we tell ourselves, but Duffles and Wild Kitty love to eat. Wild Kitty is a chef's cat, and Duffles' day consists of eating only interrupted by naps, so Delilah is the only kitty I can manage confidently.

Gatsby walks me so no problem there.

I still have poor balance, so I have no idea how I will manage getting these chonky cats into this hotel room, which, despite the weird energy from the desk lady, isn't a bad room. I start with the heaviest.

Duffles Marie!

COMING IN AT JUST OVER 20 POUNDS, SUZANNE NEEDS BOTH HANDS AND SERIOUS QUADS TO GET THIS CAT ANYWHERE.

Wild Kitty!

AT 18 POUNDS AND FULL OF FLUFF AND VENOM, SUZANNE NEARLY TRIPS WHILE GETTING HER IN THE DAYS INN!

Delilah "Blinky" Samples!

DON'T LET HER 11 POUNDS FOOL YOU—SHE WILL SCAMPER AROUND IN THE CRATE, MAKING IT NEARLY IMPOSSIBLE FOR HER MOM TO GET HER INSIDE!

Once everyone is secure in the little hotel room, I return for the supplies.

I somehow tear and spill an entire bag of cat litter by the hotel's side door.

I scurry to clean up the mess. I am exhausted from the drive, but I am not a person who mistreats hotel janitorial staff, especially during a global pandemic, dammit. I grab a plastic cup and scoop all of the wayward cat litter back into the ripped bag. I might vomit straight into the litter, and I wonder if the litter will accommodate this mishap.

I have to stop for people coming into the door. I hold it open for them as if I work for the hotel and am not feverishly scooping spilled cat litter into a giant, ripped bag.

Hi, how are you? Welcome to the Days Inn Waterloo.

I am the friendliest person in Waterloo, and I don't even have any face tattoos or drugs in me.

No matter how hard I try, I can't get that last little bit of litter into that bag, so I give up and head in for the night.

Only then do I notice I've been on camera the whole time.

I give a small curtsey and head inside.

I hope my performance has given someone at the desk some entertainment.

I guess because she associates them with luxury and comfort, Duffles absolutely loves hotels, so she bounds out of her crate and heads for the cozy bed, promptly curling up on a pillow and falling asleep. The other two are not happy; for all of their bravado at home, Delilah and Wild Kitty look like terrified kittens stranded by the side of the road. Delilah won't come out of her crate. Wild Kitty does, but she looks like she is going to cry.

I've never seen a cat look so scared.

Of course, her dad isn't here, so I do what I can to comfort her, but my anxiety is also out of control, and Wild Kitty senses this. Her gray and white fur stands on end while her green eyes continue to grieve.

What if Jeramy gets hit on the side of the road? What if the Penske People never show up, and he's there all freaking night? What if one of the Waterloo Face Tattoo people drive off the interstate with their scooter and knife him in the gut?

I listen to way too much true crime.

I remind myself Jeramy is a super capable man who can take care of himself.

I DoorDash some Chinese food.

It's the most awful tofu I've ever tried to eat.

Completely swimming in a pond of Waterloo sink water and unnamed spices, I try to take a bite of the bean curd and nearly gag. Despite the high reviews on DoorDash, this tofu belongs in the toilet.

One look at Jeramy's orange chicken tells me that the meat likely came from a hormone-addled fowl with its own tattooed neck from the side of the backwoods Waterloo highway.

Jeramy arrives at the hotel at 2 a.m. I am drugged with ibuprofen P.M. and have four animals on my bed.

Orange chicken, I say, pointing to the mini fridge. *Don't eat. Glad you're...alive, yeah.*

The phone rings at 5:30 a.m.

We let it ring.

It happens again.

Why do landline phones exist anymore?

Fuck.

I have no idea what time zone we're in right now.

Where is Waterloo?

The phone keeps ringing.

I might be dead.

Finally, Jeramy answers.

I can hear the same woman who checked me in last night screaming at Jeramy.

Oh god. Is this about the cat litter? It's got to be. I fucked up. They saw me bowing ceremoniously on camera, and now they are pissed.

I KNOW I TOLD YOU IT WAS OKAY TO PARK YOUR CAR AND TRAILER THERE BUT IT'S ACTUALLY OWNED BY THE CAR DEALERSHIP AND YOU HAVE TO MOVE IT RIGHT NOW.

Jeramy grumbles, throws on some pants, and ambles out the door. I can hear the car dealership guy fussing at him.

What made you think you could park that here? Are you serious?

The hotel told me I could.

Jeramy says he snaps under pressure sometimes, and I'm waiting.

Toilet water tofu in Waterloo.

I'm waiting.

Everywhere throughout the Greater Midwest

WALL DRUG STORE
occasional prairie dog
WALL DRUG STORE
gas station
different gas station, maybe
WALL DRUG STORE

Rapid City, South Dakota

I don't know why, but I've always wanted to see Mt. Rushmore. It's just kind of an American oddity: four presidents carved into a giant rock, potentially with an unfinished hidden tunnel inside, and you know how I feel about tunnels.

I also think of my father, who would follow this route to visit his brother in Montana. I've always wanted to be like Young Ted, wild and free, but I am much more like Old Ted, hoarding my mess into little piles everywhere, my quirkiness driving everyone crazy.

Jeramy decides to stay at the hotel with the pets, so I go alone. I get there early, before the crowds, and have no idea what to expect. There's a bit of a hike (I'm glad I have some mobility), and then there they are: Washington, Jefferson, Roosevelt, and Lincoln.

It's hard to look at those four faces and not think of the losses the Lakota Sioux suffered, but I do the American tourist thing anyway and take a selfie with the presidents. I later post the picture to social media with the caption: "Millions of peaches, peaches for free."[1]

If you know, you know.

* * *

Later that night, we eat at a Mongolian grill.

The owner, who has Taiwanese news on at volume level 100, seems annoyed Jeramy, me, and two other people have decided to eat at his restaurant. We prepare our plates (I choose mushrooms, pineapple, and tubu,[2] as it is written on the menu) and wait as the owner grills the food, never taking his eyes off the news.

I ascertain from the broadcast that someone is mad a scooter knocked over a cart of apples. A child begins to wildly throw the apples during the segment, laughing heinously in the background.

The owner gives to-go boxes to the mother and daughter who came in after us, and they open up the boxes before they pay.

I, uh, don't think these belong to us, the mom says.

YOU ORDER THIS! the owner screams at volume 100.

But this isn't ours.

YOU GET WHAT YOU GET! YOU EAT THIS NOW!

The woman tilts her head. She and her daughter exit the restaurant.

Jeramy and I laugh wildly in the background, neither of us eating the food in front of us.

Somewhere in Wyoming

I am thrilled to drive through Wyoming.

I have always wanted to be here.

Not live here or visit here, just be here.

I put Dwight Yoakam's "A Thousand Miles from Nowhere" on repeat.

Really, is there any other song to listen to when you're driving through Wyoming?

I am flummoxed Wyoming belongs to the United States. It looks like nothing I've seen here before. Really, Wyoming looks like...nothing. This vast wasteland startles me and gives me hope.

I am beginning again.

How many times have I tried to start over?

No one will know I have cancer.

No one will know how much I've struggled in the past.

No one will know how much Dwight Yoakam I've listened to.

Well, that's something I'm not ashamed of.

I remember a conversation I had with Josh about starting over. *I don't believe it's possible,* he said, confident in his words. I see what he meant, but I had to disagree. Of course it's possible! I've started over at least eight times in my life, and I'm working on number nine. True, I can't forget all my past experiences, the mistakes I made, and what I did wrong, but I wouldn't want to.

And then, in the vast nothingness people have written so many songs about, it almost happens.

My tiny car nearly smashes an antelope.

At first, I convince myself I am hallucinating.

After all, we've driven hundreds of miles and for days now, have seen nothing but flatlands, wind turbines, and Wall Drug Store billboards, which my cousin Meg warned me about. *Get ready for the Wall Drug Store billboards! You're gonna see them EVERYWHERE.*

Also, I kind of thought the whole *where the deer and antelope play* line was merely a figure of speech, an image, kind of like the whole *Columbus discovering America* thing. I didn't think pronghorn antelope actually existed in America.[3]

Well, they do in the flatlands of Wyoming, especially right in front of people's cars, and I am here to tell you all about it.

He is kind of a cute little guy, furry like a stuffed animal and with antlers pointing straight up instead of out into the woods like a deer.

I'm so glad I didn't hit it—for one, I would have been devastated if I injured or killed the one living thing Jeramy and I have seen so far in Wyoming, and for two, something as small as a pronghorn antelope would have destroyed my car.

Were they dumber than deer?

I don't know.

Maybe the pronghorn just liked taking risks.

We were the only vehicles on the road—definitely a *Twilight Zone* scenario—and the little guy pranced directly in front of me, danced a little jig, and then went on his merry way.

Because of the raised speed limits (I was born to drive out West!), I had difficulty stopping, but I managed to leave some black streaks on the open road and save all of our lives.

Jeramy drives on, missing the whole debacle entirely.

I'm 1,000 miles from nowhere, and time feels like it should matter but doesn't. I feel dizzy, but it's got to be because I'm not accustomed to all this flat terrain and immeasurable sky.

I haven't seen a pronghorn since.

Billings, Montana

At the Billings, Montana Motel 6, I see a teenager with an electronic ankle bracelet passing children out a first-floor window.

No one else seems concerned by this, but I snap a quick picture of the Missouri license plate on the van I see an adult tossing the kids into. I've seen way too many true crime shows to know you just don't let something like this go.

This Motel 6 looked fine online.

Everything looked clean and ready.

Yes, it is a Motel 6, and yes, it is only $60 a night, but I assure Jeramy everything will be fine. It's one of the only hotels in Billings, Montana, that's cat friendly, and honestly, I'm tired of everyone telling us we can't bring our cats inside after promising us on the phone it will be fine.

I'd always thought of Montana as this magical, mystical place; Mr. Samples would tell me about the *big blue skies and best fishing ever*, but so far, all we'd seen of Montana was 100-degree weather and now a Motel 6 smelling of pinto beans and burned cornbread on every floor.

The elevator is also broken.

I can manage steps most of the time, but I'm tired and starting to find myself over this trip.

We get the cats in the room, and Gatsby searches for the pinto beans and cornbread. Saddened she can't find the food, she whines as people argue in the hallway.

I done told you I ain't the father, but you wouldn't fucking believe me. This is bullshit, Mary. I done told you I wasn't his daddy.

This seems like more of a boarding house than a hotel, and I regret the decision to stay here more than ever. I make up an excuse to go outside (*I need to get that gas station fruit out of my car*), and when I get back, I see Jeramy illuminating a bedbug under the mattress.

They left the light on for us, but they also left a few roaches.

I look at Jeramy and know what to do.

I return both keys to the front desk.

You know, we had an emergency and just can't stay.

The woman raises her painted-on eyebrows.

Keep the $60, I tell her, knowing full well I will get that money back from the third-party service I used to book the hotel once I mention *bedbugs*.

Okay then! she says, and we find a hotel down the road that doesn't smell like pinto beans or burned cornbread. It's already dark, so we sneak the cats in through a side door with no cameras and fail to mention them to the front desk.

We sleep peacefully that night.

Missoula, Montana

The kid at the front desk tells me *yes, they are a pet friendly hotel, but because I didn't choose a room that was specifically pet friendly,* we cannot stay there tonight.

I'm done.

I've had it.

The kid, who looks like he has crumbs from six toaster pastries all over his face, really just wants to flirt with the blonde lady who was talking him up before I interrupted. I'm going to get nowhere because his attention is still with her, so I say JUST CANCEL IT and leave in a flurry. I sit on a bench beside a woman nodding off from what I imagine is a heroin overdose. Though I'm usually a compassionate and caring person and would ask if she was okay, I just can't do it right now.

This trip has done me in.

Her chin hits her chest, and I want to cry but can't.

I'm too tired.

Some fraternity brothers wander past us and ask if I'm going to the casino tonight.

I stare right through them as if they are part of my nationwide paranormal investigation.

Jeramy is doing something with the Penske in a semi parking lot, and it's taking forever. I let my mind wander to the lie he told me about meeting his friend for lunch. Why would he construct a lie like that? What was the point? I was out with Travis that day and told the truth, so what would be so hard about him saying, *I'm meeting my old friend Courtney for lunch.* Instead, he had to say her fiancé was there when he wasn't.

Could I trust Jeramy?

Here I was moving across the country with someone I might not be able to trust.

What the hell was I even doing?

At this point, I didn't know.

I just want to find a place to sleep.

I look up at the big sky.

The addict snorts beside me.

I'm grateful she's alive.

I'm grateful I'm alive.

The thirteenth hotel I call will give us a room for the night.

I head there with the animals and crawl into bed after opening the crates and setting up a litter box.

I am too tired for dinner or thinking or wondering or crying.

Somewhere in Idaho, I don't know

I never imagined rural life outside of West Virginia; I naively believed Appalachia was *as backwoods as it could get*, so I'm surprised to find myself in a clown car with three cats and a tired dog on the side of a very dark mountain with no cellphone service somewhere in the crooked lands of Idaho. I just expected everywhere outside of West Virginia to somehow be less rural, less backwoods, less—redneck—although deep inside of me I knew it couldn't be true.

It just couldn't be.

I was right.

I haven't seen another car for at least a hundred miles, and it's not even 9 p.m. yet. I could drive all the way to Pullman (our final destination) tonight, but Jeramy has the key code to

239

our new place, and I can't get in touch with him. I have no idea if he will have phone service at all now or even tomorrow.

The last I heard, he was sleeping at a truck stop.

He needed to get a new cell phone.

Or something.

I don't even know.

Somehow after sleeping at the same hotel last night, we got separated between Montana and Idaho.

As narrated by Keith Morrison: *Jeramy was last in touch with his girlfriend before they parted ways three hours outside Coeur d'Alene, Idaho. The couple was moving to Washington for a fresh start. A new life. Jeramy's phone, completely out of service with no hope of returning, last sent Suzanne a message near the Montana border telling her to head to Idaho with their pets, and he would meet her there. Only one of them would arrive.*

I'm about to run out of gas, and there are no signs for any stations.

This is worse than West Virginia, though fewer deer. There are at least signs for gas stations in WV, even if they don't exist once you pull off the exit.

The setting sun casts an eerie cerise light through the Western Hemlocks, obscuring my view of anything past the mountain. I expect a Sasquatch family or UFO to greet me at any moment; I can't say I would mind. With the animals all crashed, I'm feeling pretty lonely and terrified on this drive.

Honestly, if I weren't a West Virginia driver, comfortable with roads curvier than a good hillbilly woman, I'd be so fucked.

Although I don't have cell service, I hope for the best and shoot Emily a text.

Missing 411 Idaho.

She will know what it means.

I start to wonder if I'm already dead and actually driving through the afterlife.

I am suddenly confused about the time of day and can't tell if it's twilight, dawn, or some odd time in the middle of the night when all my devices have broken down and left me timeless. I have no idea what time zone I'm actually in anymore, and although I'm hopeful I'll reach Coeur d'Alene before pure darkness hits, I can't tell if it will actually happen or not. The trees are taller here, the roads narrower.

Is that an outline of Bigfoot I see in the pines?

I hope Jeramy spends the night in Montana. There's no way he could safely make it with the Brokse in the dark on these roads.

Sure, he'd find it fun, but I can't make it on my own out here.

For the first time in my life, I feel like I actually need someone.

I start hallucinating UFOs in the pink sky, oblong little shits that will carry me away to another planet...or maybe I have already joined their planet? Seriously, why are there no other cars on this road? Where the fuck am I? Sure, my GPS quit working about an hour ago, but there was no other place to go.

I am going to run out of gas.

I do not have service.

Jeramy is in another state, having coffee at a goddamn truck stop.

I am going to be on the side of the road with four dehydrated animals, most likely on another planet where no one but maybe Emily and the guy who wrote the *Missing 411* series will know where we are.

I try to appreciate the scenery.

This!

This is what inspires artists to paint, these trees, this sky!

I have never seen these colors before.

And then, out of nowhere, a gas station.

I do not want to be fooled. I am from Appalachia, where gas stations pretend to exist. I could waste a few precious miles pulling off the exit only to find nothing there.

I take my chances.

Suddenly, any hope of seeing Sasquatch or a UFO disappears faster than Jeramy's truck stop coffee.

Am I a little disappointed about this? I am. Relieved, yes, but disappointed.

This might have been my only shot.

Coeur d'Alene, Idaho

Coeur d'Alene appears like a bright earthly village after being in an alien spaceship for a few hours. Somehow a brief period of daylight resonates in the city, and everything here is as lively as a college party.

Bigfoot is nowhere in sight, but maybe he got into the clubs. My hotel is near a few bars, but I don't mind. Though I usually prefer quiet solitude, I am comforted by the chatter of human beings surrounding us.

I put the room, which is the biggest space we've had so far, on a credit card. I feel like I deserve this.

I can only hope Jeramy is still alive out there, perhaps at a truck stop in Montana?

I can't worry about him; I have three cats to get to a fourth floor.

Once settled, Duffles sits on the bed and looks out at the city lights. Cathleen says I should write a children's book called *Hotel Duffles* and sell it with an accompanying calico plushie.

It would be a great idea if I knew how to write children's books.

It's a more specific field than most people realize.

I order pancakes from DoorDash and settle in. Pancakes are the absolute worst food for my blood sugar, but I don't care. This is the most relaxed I've felt in a long time, and I plan to enjoy myself.

After all, I was possibly abducted by aliens earlier in Idaho (how will I ever know?) and then had to drag four animals from a parking lot, into an elevator, and down a long hallway, so I feel like I deserve some sugary snacks.

I take a picture of myself in the cheval mirror, and the snapshot gives off an odd blue light.

I was definitely abducted by aliens, and things will never be the same again.

The cats, Gatsby, and I sleep well that night; Jeramy meets us in the morning. My blood sugar is high from the pancakes, and his clothes are wrinkled and smell like burnt coffee from spending the night at the truck stop.

We are almost home.

PART V
GAPS

Pullman, Washington

We park in our new driveway, and there might as well be red flags lining the concrete.

The yard is completely overgrown, and although I remember our lease saying *the tenant is responsible for yard upkeep*, it seems no one has touched this grass in three years.

Jeramy and I decide to take in an inflatable mattress for the night and get everything else in the morning.

What meets us inside is way more frightening than the overgrown yard.

Far from the spiffy house we saw online, this space hasn't been cleaned since they allowed students to rent it in 1979. The kitchen appliances? Held together with black duct tape. Like memories of drunken make out sessions, pieces of gum remain stuck to the floor from that rager Elias and Ben had two years ago. The bedroom on the left? At least three urine stains from a dog or human.

Impossible to tell, but it's definitely urine.

I find a pile of cigarette butts by the fireplace and wonder if homeless people somehow snuck in here without a key. It would explain a few mishaps but not everything.

Um didn't the landlady say she came in and checked everything last week? I ask Jeramy as I examine a spot of black mold by the washer and dryer.

Sure did, he says as he moves things about. His mom owns and rents properties that he's assisted her with, so he knows what to look for. *It has potential*, he says, but I can tell we are both thinking *no fucking way*.

The bathroom, which was sparkling blue in the pictures online, looks as if it's an old dorm shower hundreds of students have used. I eyeball a chunk of hair curled up in the corner like an animal ready to attack.

I might vomit, and I'm not even on chemo.

The one decent part of the apartment?

The ten feet of new carpet the landlady wouldn't shut up about.

Whenever we spoke with her, she kept mentioning the *new carpet*, and now I know why: It's the only part of this duplex worth mentioning.

I steady myself and wonder if perhaps the place just needs a good clean. I walk around again and realize nope. That urine is deep, decades deep, in the laminate. The smell will not come out, no matter how many times we pressure wash that floor.

So, we do what anyone else new to Washington who was just rented a scam duplex would do.

Go get some legal weed.

I am interested in a substance called Rick Simpson Oil, which is supposed to be ace for brain cancer, and Jeramy just wants something to chill him out from the hellish drive and horrendous apartment situation.

Understandable.

We find a store that was definitely an old Ponderosa restaurant, and I've already told myself Pullman is a new beginning. I don't want a soul here knowing I had (have? I ask myself) cancer. Because of this, I strut into the weed shop and announce several times I *want the best Rick Simpson Oil they have.*

According to Jeramy, what the lovely gal helping us hears is, *I want the strongest shit you've got.*

We leave the shop with our wares and head back to The Drug Den for the night. I can tell we aren't sure exactly what to do. Before we indulge in our legal products, we read our lease multiple times and believe we have found a caveat: *something something as long as the tenant does not fully move in, they have 24 hours to rescind the lease.*

We plan to meet with the landlady tomorrow afternoon, pretend we arrived tomorrow morning, and see what we can do.

But first, I follow the internet's advice, take a rice-sized amount of RSO, and try to relax.

I'm going to cure my brain cancer.

Well, except that the internet lies sometimes, and a rice-sized amount for me turns out to be about five times too much.

The night begins just fine; we release the cats from their crates and blow up a mattress Jeramy received as a gift from work. Of course, we put the mattress on *the new carpet.* The trouble starts when sweet Duffles, who lacks claw control, jumps onto the mattress and deflates the entire bed. Terrified of the sinking sensation, Duffles disappears into the urine bedroom and cries all night.

All. Night.

I've never heard her do that before.

The meowing never stops, and she won't leave the room to sleep with us.

Later, Jeramy tells me the *house is definitely haunted by something.*

Then the RSO hits.

It's nothing like the people on Instagram said. I don't experience *a calm, collected feeling I'm going to be cured.* Instead, I cry uncontrollably. I ask Jeramy if we can talk, and I just let loose with the tears. *I'm afraid I'm going to die alone and nothing is going to be okay and I don't want to do this to you and I'm so scared of everything all this cancer shit and I'm going to die soon Jeramy don't you get that and what were you thinking taking all this on with me and did you think this through and I think I might love you but that's fucking insane because I have brain cancer and it's just honestly too much for me to handle sometimes and no one ever wants to talk about it and it wears on me it really does and sometimes I just need to talk about it and no one ever wants to and I can't live like that.*

Hey, hey, Jeramy says as he hugs me close on the ten feet of new carpet. *It's always going to be you and me, Wiggles.*

He's called me Wiggles since the first weekend I stayed with him. I earned the nickname because according to him, I wiggled all the way across the bed and nearly pushed him off both nights.

It's an apt nickname.

I calm down for a moment because I know I can trust him.

And then the RSO sends me to a dark place.

Jeramy falls asleep, and The Drug Den blurs before me like I'm already dead. Gatsby blends in with the ten feet of new carpet until she melts into it like a puddle. I don't know where Delilah and Wild Kitty are, but I can still here Duffles crying in the urine room, and there's nothing I can do about it.

I cannot walk or stand.

Thanks, RSO.

I can't deal with anything in front of me, so I close my eyes and try to sleep. I can hear Jeramy snoring on the ten feet of new carpet beside me, and I know I need to do the same.

One problem: The RSO has caused me to hear a female voice in my head. She's a game show host, wearing bright primary colors. I am a contestant, but if I don't win, I die. I am losing, I am dying. I am stuck. I can't get away from the game show host. She keeps repeating the same phrases again and again.

Soap for new apartment! Ten dollars and ninety-three cents!

You can't cure your brain cancer, you know that, right?

Suzanne. Welcome to the special Rick Simpson Game Show. You are the lassssst contestant! You have managed to create your own consciousness and now you will never escape.

And then I hear Jeramy's voice in the crowd. I know if I can just find him and hang onto him, everything will be fine.

JERRY SPITLER.

Wait. Why is he saying his name is Jerry Spitler? It's close to Jeramy, but that's definitely not a nickname he has ever given himself. I try to find his voice and never let it go, but the words slip away from me like my health.

Soap for new apartment! Ten dollars and ninety-three cents!

You can't cure your brain cancer, you know that, right?

Suzanne. Welcome to the special Rick Simpson Game Show. You are the lassssst contestant! You have managed to create your own consciousness and now you will never escape.

JERRY SPITLER.

There he is again.

I try to find him in the crowd of people, but he eludes me.

The lady's voice becomes more computerized and mechanical.

Soap for new apartment. Ten dollars and ninety-three cents.

You can't cure your brain cancer, you know that, right?

Suzanne. Welcome to the special Rick Simpson Game

251

Show. You are the lassssst contestant. You have managed to create your own consciousness and now you will never escape.

JERRY SPITLER.

I try to hug his words, but it's no use. I can't reach them. I have created my own consciousness, and I cannot escape. This. This is how I will die. I am falling down a green and black hole, and Duffles cries for me.

JERRY SPITLER.

* * *

I wake up the next morning still high but definitely alive.

I'm never taking RSO again.

Fuck Instagram advice.

We dump everything back in the Penske and pretend we never stayed in The Drug Den. Jeramy walks through the place with the landlady and goes through all the ways the duplex is an absolute piece of shit. I hear her say, *But it has new carpet!* and I roll my eyes. The caveat in the lease saves us and gets our deposit back.

I also throw in a *look, I have brain cancer, and there is mold everywhere* bit, and it works.

After four days at The Quality Inn, we end up finding an apartment in a complex that's like an oversized dorm. It kinda blows, but it doesn't have mold or urine on the floor, so we make it work.

JERRY SPITLER and I are officially Pacific Northwesterners.

Seattle, Washington

I drive to my new doctor in Seattle.

It takes over four hours to get to the big city from Pullman, and there are approximately one-and-a-half gas stations. I discover this when I pull off an exit claiming to have petrol when, as it turns out, there is a singular gas pump with a free-standing debit card reader next to a field with two horses.

No building.

Just a gas pump, a diesel pump, and two horses.

There are also three cowboys parked there, shooting the shit outside of their jacked-up pickups.

Okay, I get it. It's no different from West Virginia, except for the hat size.

I hear them laughing as I attempt to figure out how to pump this fucking gas. This station is strangely anachronistic, the cowboys and horse field next to high-tech pumps and debit card reader. I figure the card reader out, pump my gas, and sit with my feet dangling from my car.

The cowboys spit in my direction.

They are around my age, which makes them seem more threatening for some reason.

I ain't never seen a car like that.

Did Robert Wadlow lose a house slipper?

Th' ell is Robert Wadlow[1]?

I need to get out of here, but I do laugh a little.

I can't help myself.

* * *

After spending the night at my pineapple-themed hotel, I am ready to meet my tumor team. I picked my hotel because it was within walking distance of the hospital.

The free pineapple cookies are an added bonus.

I walk into the Alvord Brain Tumor Center and although I tell myself this will be nothing like *Grey's Anatomy*, it's almost exactly like *Grey's Anatomy*. The hospital is giant, and everyone is perky, young, and perfectly attractive. I brought a giant backpack full of nothing but snacks.

I am assigned to The Gold Team.

My initial nurse seems way more excited about this than I do. I have no idea who The Gold Team is, but judging by her enthusiasm, The Gold Team is worth smiling about. I can see her expression through her mask.

Though this is not part of her duties, the nurse lifts my backpack and carries it into my appointment room after I am weighed.

Miss, what do you have in here? she asks.

Umm. I am very embarrassed.

Snacks? That's it. That's everything.

There's a boba smoothie, a granola bar, some cookies from the hotel, a giant bottle of water, and a turkey sandwich. I've been too nervous to eat or drink any of it, and for whatever reason, my blood sugar is over 300.

She laughs hysterically.

You can sit wherever you are comfortable, and then the nurse will see you. I might eat some of your snacks.

I am confused. I thought she was the nurse. She held all my papers, weighed me like an animal headed to slaughter, and guided me back to this fancy pod.

Oh, I mean the nurse practitioner from The Gold Team! she explains, sensing my bewilderment.

I've never been able to disguise my face. There's Resting Bitch Face, Resting Friendly Face, and then what I have, which I call Resting Can't Fucking Hide Anything Face.

Ohhh you will just love The Gold Team! They are all so good, just like an Olympic gold medal. The best. When you come back for other appointments, I'll be the regular nurse, but you'll meet the nurse practitioner from The Gold Team today. He'll get your full story, vitals, and all that good stuff.

She squeezes my hand.

I feel like I'm going to faint.

You're going to be just fine.

I meek like a cat.

The nurse practitioner enters, and although he looked pretentious on the website (I, naturally, did thorough research and thought I made a mistake when I met the earlier nurse), Nurse Brien is attentive and as interested in my specific case as a nerdy kid in advanced organic chemistry. He studies my walking patterns, facial expressions, and speech. Although someone out there might enjoy this type of attention, I'd rather be out exploring some wacky Seattle coffee shop than sitting here smiling and frowning for Nurse Brien. At least there is no MRI today, no needles, and no results to fret over. Surprisingly, Nurse Brien seems as kind as my care team in The Dash. Although Winston-Salem is a city by North Carolina standards, I feared that I would become a dreaded number in Seattle, just another patient in the DMV of cancer care waiting to be called to the nurse's station and shuffled through the line before the end of the day.

However, Nurse Brien actually asks me to tell him my story, which I somehow condense into a brief paragraph. *I was at a coffee shop one morning, and I thought I was experiencing a Charley Horse. It kept going up my leg and into my shoulder, and I realized I was having a seizure and was paralyzed on my right side. I went to the ER, they told me I had a mass on my brain, they transported me to a bigger hospital, and then I had a craniotomy right before Christmas of 2017. I did a bunch of physical therapy, learned to walk again, and sadly learned the tumor was glioblastoma. I did temozolomide chemo and radiation...and years later, here I am?*

Nurse Brien listens and takes notes.

I need a nap.

Thank you so much for telling me everything. The doctor will be in to see you soon, and I will update her before she sees you so you don't have to go through all of this again, okay?

Thank goodness.

I am a bit confused, though. Typically, in my experience, whenever you see a nurse practitioner, this means you won't be seeing the doctor. I think I am off the hook, but nope, I guess not.

The Gold Team has standards.

Atomic standards.

Before I can even dig into my snack pack, Dr. McG breezes into the room with her cadre of medical scribes.

Hi! I'm Dr. McG, and these lovely people—she gestures broadly to four folks who might be teenagers or twentysomethings who would rather be skateboarding than recording neurological symptoms—*will be taking some notes for me today, if that's okay with you.*

Of course, I say, but honestly, I would say anything right now. I am already in awe of Dr. McG. I assume, and my later research confirms, she is around my age, my age exactly, a neuro-oncologist, a professor at the hospital's adjoining University of Washington, and looks like a freaking Barbie doll.

For real.

Without even trying, this woman wakes up and looks gorgeous.

I can tell within our first interaction, Dr. McG is nice. Tough but nice. I admire her

at once. I want to be her, except I seriously wonder how much sleep she gets at night.

She quickly goes over what Nurse Brien briefed her on, does a quick overview of my neurological symptoms, and then says, *I hear you're often unsure of how to tell the difference between diabetes issues and neurological symptoms.*

I am overwhelmed by how television this all seems, and I'm having trouble concentrating because I can't wait to tell what friends I have left about how surreal this is.

Always, I stammer. *It's...it's sometimes hard to tell. And... I've been having dizzy spells. It could be from moving to a new climate. It could be fatigue. It could be sinus trouble.* I realize with absolute horror I sound, in this moment, just like my mom. Everything—my brain tumor, her stroke, the first moon landing —was actually a sinus infection. I don't tell Dr. McG that sometimes when I wake up in the morning, my head feels like it's going to roll off my body. How do you say those words to a doctor in absolute seriousness? Sure, that's how it feels, but what's the medical terminology for *my head feels like it's rolling off my body when I wake up in the morning?* I'm afraid I'll open my eyes and make direct contact with one of my cats on the floor while my body hangs in bed?

So, I go with *I've been having dizzy spells.*

Okay, she tells me as she shines a light into my eye. *That doesn't worry me right off the bat.*

I breathe six months of anxiety away. If these dizzy spells don't concern Dr. McBarbie (and I write that with utmost respect and not sarcasm—she's gorgeous), then I am not worried either.

I do want you to have MRIs every three months, though.

And there's my Resting Can't Fucking Hide Anything Face again.

You don't look too happy about that.

Dr. McBarbie can even read people. There's nothing, absolutely nothing this woman can't do.

She is a Seattle pillar. She should have a hospital wing named after her, or at least a bench in the commons. She is a goddess.

Yeah, I hate them, like everyone else, I'm sure.

257

Okay, every four months then.

She can debate. She can compromise. She can do everything.

I bet she volunteers on the weekends.

I leave the office in a bit of a tailspin. I take an expensive Uber back to my boutique pineapple hotel, dig through my backpack for my boba smoothie (which is slightly warm but whatever), and rinse out the plastic bottle, deciding to save it because the cat on it looks exactly like Duffles, and I miss her.

I miss home.

Pullman is not everything Jeramy and I imagined it might be—it's a strange mishmash of drunk college kids, wheat, soybeans, and desert— but he and the animals comprise my entire world now, and I like it that way. Suddenly, I have everything I could have ever wanted. Sure, it took forty years, too much school, a marriage that feels like it didn't even happen, ten years of dating women, and a brain cancer diagnosis, but I'm finally happy, or something close to that.

But first.

I have some old business to take care of.

* * *

Nodya "Paina Skully" Boyko and I have to fuck some shit up in Seattle.

When Auburn accepted me into grad school, I didn't have the means to visit beforehand and secure a proper apartment. The English department had misplaced my acceptance letter (it fell behind a file cabinet in the main office), and if I hadn't called, they might have assumed I turned down full funding into the Ph.D. lit program.

I didn't realize how small Auburn is, and I just assumed I could find an apartment at a moment's notice. I loaded my kitty

Pru and some clothes into my Subaru and hoped for the best on the 13-hour drive from Harrisville, West Virginia, to Auburn, Alabama. Every call I made along the way ended with *sorry, nothing is available.*

At a rest stop in rural South Carolina, I found a pet-friendly apartment complex in Opelika, Alabama, which, according to my rusty flip phone, wasn't too far from Auburn. I took an agitated breath and called.

Welllll, the manager said with a molasses Southern drawl, *we did have one unit left, but a gal from Seattle with a blind cat called about five minutes ago and rented it out.*

Dammit.

That girl was Nodya "Paina Skully" Boyko, and she would later become one of my very best friends.

I ended up renting a trailer full of cockroaches with a floor that fell through in the winter, but it built character.

Skully and I bonded over our love of *The Office* (before it was cool), our snarky sense of humor, and similar social values. Although we both maintained our model student status and received the highest marks, we were also fond of country karaoke at a redneck bar in Opelika called Jackie Lee's, where, if the crowd was lucky, the eponymous owner (a Black cowboy), would appear and serenade everyone with a country classic or two.

One night, we somehow started at Jackie Lee's and ended up at an undergrad bar with a hipster and a local who looked like Bobcat Goldthwait, all of us onstage belting out Outkast's "So Fresh, So Clean," though none of us really knew the words.

Afterward, I Irish exited and walked home, leaving Skully to deal with Bobcat and the hipster by herself.

Auburn has never been the same since.

After our grad school stint in Alabama, we have followed

one another around the country, playing roller derby and generally getting into shenanigans.

In Seattle, we tear up some shopping at a store where two hipsters sew something strange in the corner, buy some lotion bars at Pike Place Market, and take a picture with Rachel the bronze pig.

It's the last time all three of us will be smiling.

Pullman, Washington

Back home, Jeramy leaves for work, and I need to write.

I want to use YouTube to listen to music.

I can't think of a single band I like.

Am I losing myself in this relationship?

Am I forgetting who I am?

Have I become, Fogwoman forbid, a *moldable girlfriend*?

No.

Something is wrong something is wrong something is wrong.

Pullman, Washington

I completely stop feeling like myself toward the end of summer.

A break here, a snap there.

I am mad about everything.

I need to go to bed at 7 p.m.

I am dizzy all the time.

I don't know how much longer I can wake up feeling like this.

The nausea the sleeplessness the grand irritation of it all.

. . .

Pullman, Washington

Jeramy and I decide to go fishing, but we need to stop for bait first. Perhaps not surprisingly, I am a decent fisherwoman. My dad loves fishing, and I am a natural (except when I have to take the fish off the hook, then I scream), which is great because I desperately needed a new hobby.

When Jeramy isn't looking, I always throw one worm back into the dirt and tell myself I am saving a life.

By the bait section, I receive an email: I have a message in MyChart notifying me I have a new test result. This can't be right. I haven't had any tests yet. I'm a brand-new patient and have only had a meet-and-greet appointment.

This must be a mistake.

I quickly pull up the results.

Overall, the combined histomorphological and molecular features of the current specimen are most supportive of a *high-grade astrocytoma with piloid features* (which has also been referred to as anaplastic astrocytoma with piloid features). This entity is a relatively newly categorized IDH-wild-type astrocytoma which often harbors MAPK pathway gene mutations, homozygous deletion of CDKN2A/B and loss of ATRX expression [1-3].

I scan the rest of the document and ascertain that my tumor, now four years old, has been retested by the lab in Seattle, and I feel the store spin around me in a tie-dye of fluorescent hunting gear and camouflage tents. (We are in Idaho, after all.) I grab onto the fridge of worms where Jeramy searches for nightcrawlers.

Are you okay? he asks.

No. No I am not. What the hell is this? What is happening? I assumed my tumor was tossed out into some biohazard

261

container after the original biopsy and never seen or heard from again. Maybe some rabid coyotes ate it or something. *Where has it been hiding?* What does this mean? What the hell is a *high-grade astrocytoma with piloid features?* Is this really my tumor?

I don't have glioblastoma?

I've spent the last four years believing I had something I didn't?

Hell, I wrote two books about something I don't have?

IS ANYONE GOING TO TALK TO ME ABOUT THIS?

My brain, the working parts of it anyway, starts going wild. How could they do this without informing me? Shouldn't they ask before retesting my tumor? How much is this going to cost?

I'm about to shit my pants.

I follow Jeramy to the car. I tell him what's happening, but he doesn't see the big deal. He's more concerned about the upcoming fishing trip.

This is kind of important, I tell him. *I'm basically getting a new diagnosis, different from what I've had the past four years, and I don't know why I'm getting it. No one told me they were doing it, I don't know who is paying for it, and I don't know what it means.*

I frantically Google *high grade astrocytoma with piloid features* and one scholarly article appears.

One.

No Wikipedia page.

Nothing from the World Health Organization, though I understand because they've been rather busy these past couple years.

Jeramy doesn't seem supportive right now, so I read the one article I found. It's a rather short study and doesn't tell me a whole lot. This report details five people diagnosed with high grade astrocytomas with piloid features or HGAPs. At the time of the study, three died, one was doing fine, and one stop returning the study's calls and inquiries.

And that's all I get.

It seems HGAPs aren't so different from glioblastomas but are a rare combo of piliod tumors and astrocytomas. Theoretically, I could have had the piliod tumor since I was a kid because they are most often diagnosed in children. Then the astrocytoma part, I'm guessing, grew later. At this point in the car I'm only speculating, and I'm not sure what is happening right now. I'm upset the doctor's office didn't even tell me about the tumor testing.

Jeramy doesn't care about anything but the fishing trip.

I feel lonelier than I have in a long time.

* * *

I catch seven trout that day.

I watch the fog settle over the lake and smother the surface.

One of the fish I threw back gurgles to the surface, dead.

I know I am in trouble.

Nowhere

I am drawing a blank I am drawing a blank I am drawing a blank and this is how I know something is wrong something is wrong something is wrong but I don't want to admit it to myself or Jeramy or anyone else and I'm not sure anyone would believe me but I am drawing a blank a big blank and I am worried very worried and so scared I am right because I haven't drawn a blank since this happened last time and I'm not the type of person to draw a blank especially about stuff I know but I can't think of any of the *Jeopardy!* questions tonight even though there is a category about Victorian Lit and I can't even remember Charles Goddamn Dickens and that's how I know for sure something is very wrong.

Something is very wrong.

Seattle, Washington

I am stuffed with pineapple cookies and ready for this MRI.

After a gorgeous, rainy walk to the hospital from the citrus-themed hotel, I feel like nothing could go wrong. I'm in a trustworthy hospital with intelligent people. This MRI should be easy.

I should know better by now.

Five hours later I've had:

- Four people try to find a good vein, including:
- Two nurses
- Two doctors from the anesthesia team
- One ultrasound machine
- Three French Hens
- Four shots of lidocaine
- Ten attempts at an IV
- One IV flush that caused the two MRI techs to go into a complete panic and cover my arm with a cloth so I didn't have to see (and so they didn't have to see it, if I had to guess) my arm swelling to the size of a water balloon[2]
- And a partridge in a pear tree!

(It's September, so you know it's close enough for Christmas music.)

. . .

When traditional methods fail, they decide to do an ultrasound IV. Dr. Maria, the first doctor they send, can't stand too close to the MRI machines because she is too magnetically kind. She holds my arm gently before injecting the lidocaine, which I love because then I can't feel her digging around in there and searching for my invisible veins. I can tell she frustrates herself and is not accustomed to screwing up, but she tries not to let me see her disappointment. She takes cell phone breaks to check on her patients.

Hello, this is Mare-eeah. Yes, okay. She is doing fine then. Okay. Okay.

She comes back to holding my arm with her warm hand and says, *We always say our nicest patients get cancer. It's just not fair. It's always the nice ones.*

I want to tell her I am not nice all the time, but it's not her fault she can't get my IV in. My blood vessels are complete shit and seem to disappear as soon as the needle pops into my skin.

I have forgotten: This is a teaching hospital.

Although Maria might be the nicest anesthesiologist ever, she's not great at this IV business. Finally, an anesthesiologist dude bro comes into my curtained area, stabs me quickly, and it's done.

I'm not really a fan of dude bros, but I am when they get the job done.

The MRI, after the IV business, happens relatively fast, and then I rush upstairs. I haven't eaten since the morning cookies, and I didn't bring my snack backpack this time.

It's Friday, naturally, and it's 5:30 p.m. before I get to my appointment. There is no nurse and no vitals. I don't even care about the results anymore. Well, I do. I just want to know and get back to the hotel.

Dr. McBarbie rushes in, still looking put together and like she just accepted an Emmy.

What the hell happened?

I am really bad at getting IVs, I say, and then we don't waste any time.

Okay, we have some stuff to discuss. We retest all our new patient's tumors, Dr. McBarbie says. *I'm sorry we didn't tell you. That must have been a shock to see all that come up in MyChart and have no idea what was happening.*

It certainly was, I say.

I can see Dr. McBarbie's blue eyes flash with excitement.

So, what you have—a High Grade Astrocytoma with Piloid features—is exceedingly rare. I really couldn't believe it when I saw the results.

I don't want to be exceedingly rare, I say, and no one knows how to respond.

Oh, she is pumped. I've never seen a doctor so excited. I can tell she's trying to contain herself, but she just can't.

This might be her once in a lifetime brain tumor.

The World Health Organization hasn't even come out with this specific designation yet, but they will soon. It's very rare. There aren't many of you out there. Exceedingly rare, my dear.

I feel like I'm living in a sci-fi novel.

Which makes what I'm about to tell you less scary, perhaps.

I knew it.

Some areas of concern showed up on the MRI that...we aren't sure about. They could be new tumors, or they could be radiation necrosis. Some of them...I've never quite seen anything like this.

Baffled, she cocks her head.

Dr. McBarbie brings up the MRI to show me. There is one major spot I see on the right side of my brain, and several smaller *areas of concern* on the left side.

My brain is a tunnel, and there are many explorers who have turned on their headlamps.

266

I'm not sure why she's never seen anything like them except that she's never had a patient with HGAP tumors before.

I am extremely overwhelmed I am extremely overwhelmed I am extremely overwhelmed.

Are you okay? she asks.

Fine, yeah, totally good.

The reason I have hope, she tells me, *is because* (she pauses to take out a pencil and piece of paper to draw a diagram) *glioblastomas grow outward and HGAPs grow inward. So, I want to do another MRI in four weeks and see what's happening. If there's growth, we will discuss what to do next. If these areas stay the same, we can assume it's radiation necrosis.*

I understand.

I am not in shock. I expected this.

How are you feeling? she asks.

I expected this. I mean, it's not good, but I'm okay.

I am not okay.

I'm worried about you. Are you alone tonight?

No, I lie.

I leave the office and head out into the Seattle night, Sufjan Stevens "Should Have Known Better" on my Spotify, not sure what to feel or say to anyone.

I don't say anything.

Pullman, Washington

We've been fighting a lot, Jeramy says. He sighs. He's frustrated. He's probably going to leave me.

I don't respond. I don't know how to. Yeah, we have been fighting a lot. I sit in this apartment complex all day, surrounded by college students at a university where I don't teach and don't have an opportunity to. The steroid junkie above us emotionally abuses his girlfriend all day and night by screaming at her loud enough for all of building H to hear, and she responds by stomping like a baby elephant.

Don't get me wrong—I feel for her. I met her while doing laundry, and she's smart and sweet and I want her to get the hell out of there, but her constant mud spraying is not helpful to the ever-frequent headaches I'm experiencing. I'm sitting here at this apartment responding to student emails, questions I've already answered at least three times before, all while trying to reduce my screen time so my eyes don't roll back into my rotting brain.

I don't know how I'm doing any of this, quite honestly.

All the while I don't know if I have active cancer again or not.

Jeramy is gone all day, working hard but also having conversations and meeting people and cutting up with friends at work, taking *safety breaks*[3] with pretty girls and sharing the coffee I buy with his work buddies, although he makes a ton more money than I do.

Jeramy apologizes, says he understands why I feel this way.

He promises to do better. I believe him. He feels attacked and says I am mean.

It's in your tone, he says.

He is not wrong.

The other day when I told him he wasn't emotionally available after his other live-in relationship didn't work out, I said, *That must have been the most bomb ass pussy on the planet because even though it was a decade ago, you sure can't seem to be happy with anyone else's.* Was it mean? Yes. Was it also slightly funny? On some level, yes, I would like to think so.

I think of Cathleen, who looks like a Kardashian version of myself and always says, *I love being mean. It's my brand. If I'm not mean to a man, something is wrong. I want to be known for being mean.* I get the uncontrollable giggles whenever I think of this. I've always had the same problem, but this time, I feel guilty being mean. It's the easy way out, and I've done it for too long.

I don't want to be mean to him.

I also don't want him giving my (potential, if it's truly back) cancer time to other people he'll have plenty of time with later.

I wonder about this far too often.

I am dying.

He says I'm too worried about what I don't know.

Jeramy and I are the same age; he's exactly 20 days older than I am.

We are both about to turn 40, and I am doubtful I will make it to 41.

Barring a tragic accident or serious health issue of his own, Jeramy still has half his life ahead of him, and it would be ridiculous of me to assume he's not going to be with anyone else after I'm gone. I've noticed, in my casual observances, men tend to move on pretty quickly, and yeah, I'll be dead, but who will he move on with? What will she look like? Will he have a string of casual relationships, develop a cocaine habit he doesn't have now, and have a bunch of drug-fueled one-night stands with busty brunettes who, only in a certain damp hotel light, remind him of me? Or will he jump into a serious relationship with a tall blonde who loves cooking and pet mice but hates the word *fuck*? She would be quite the opposite of me, but maybe that's what he would need.

I mean, I'm going to haunt them either way, just a kitchen drawer opens here, a light switching on and off there, little brief reminders I'm never going away.

I know this shouldn't matter, but I can't help but think of it. I can't be one of those *Chicken Soup for the Soul* stories where I find a suitable partner for my boyfriend before I go. He will be just fine on his own for a minute or two.

I would never want him to be unhappy, but I can't stomach the thought of him being with someone else. I don't care about him fucking someone else once I'm a trillion ashes stuffed away behind The Owl Picture in Emily's living room, but I feel more nauseated than when I'm on chemo about him giving someone else a nickname like *Wiggles* or making another girl a kitty cat nest in bed like he makes for me.

I don't think I'll ever get over this, even when I'm taking my last breath.

A distant land in Idaho

Despite my current situation, Jeramy thinks I should go camping in Idaho.

Alone.

He's busy cooking for the semester, but it will be the last chance to camp for the season. He thinks it will *give me back some feelings of independence*, and I agree.

Once I arrive at the campsite, I help a former child star from India with his fire, and he helps me set up my tent.

Everything is fine until I decide to venture *to town* for some snacks and end up circling around an Idaho mountain. I lose signal and with no place to turn around, must continue up the dirt road hairpin turns, switchbacking on the steep incline until I reach the summit and can circle back down.

I am on an ATV trail.

Boulders mar the already narrow roads; my knuckles match the eggplant shade of my tiny Scion, and I know if I was in any other car, I wouldn't have made it.

I'm still not sure I did.

The Ponderosa Pines and Grand Firs wave to me with delight. I'm certain they haven't seen a person in decades.

If this isn't a metaphor for the last four years, I don't know what is.

Seattle, Washington

I don't know why I'm having this MRI. I already know the results. It's more of a *let's make sure of this* situation for Dr. McBarbie, but I don't have any expectations of the two magic words: radiation necrosis.

At least the MRI was easier this time; they remembered.

A quick lidocaine pop in my right arm, the one with *the good vein, the only good vein she has*, and I am ready for the test.

I request 2010s *Indie* as the listening companion for my MRI, and the tech raises an eyebrow at the specificity but complies.

I like what I like.

As Father John Misty bleeds into my ears (I've come around to him lately), time slows to an uncomfortable, slushed pace. The tempo of the song stretches into *reaaaaaaal luuuuu-uvvvvvv babbbbbbeeeeee ooooohhhh*, and I feel the cool metallic taste of the gadolinium contrast numb my mouth and slide into my brain.

I know.

I know.

I know something is for sure wrong, very wrong.

I had suspected something was wrong when my hand felt strange, when Jeramy and I moved across the country, even back when I was having suicidal ideations in the Charleston hotel, and I started having dizzy spells. Everyone told me, I told

271

myself *there is no reason to be concerned,* but there was a reason to be concerned.

A major reason.

I wonder now why no one listened to me.

* * *

Dr. McBarbie glides into the pod and asks me how I feel.

Anxious, I say.

Uh oh. She doesn't stick to her usual style of padding everything with a little bit of conversation.

I am right I am right I am right.

Well, I'm going to pull up these images, but...I'm afraid I can't ease your anxiety much.

Unlike 2017 when I thought I was cancer free and was told I had glioblastoma, this news does not send me feeling like I'm falling through the floor. My feet stay as firmly planted as the old oaks by the tunnels I explored last summer.

As she reveals the MRI, I can see the *area of concern* on my right side has grown—not exponentially, but some, like an acorn dropped into mud.

So, this definitely isn't radiation necrosis. These other spots, though, she says as I detect absolute bafflement in her voice, *well, some of them have just...disappeared, which I truly don't understand. You are something else.*

I don't care about the disappearing spots. Cool, sure, but I want to know what to do about the acorn.

What are we going to do?

My Resting Can't Fucking Hide Anything Face has left the building. I don't know who this completely expressionless person who sits in front of Dr. McBarbie is. I have zero emotion.

None.

Well, we can start you on chemo. It would be another pill but different than temozolomide. Or we can wait.

I want the chemo, I say without pause.

I know.

I know I wrote in my last book I *wasn't going to do anything else.* Now my life is better. My life has changed. I have a new cat, a boyfriend, live in a new area, and have a literary magazine to run.

I need this chemo.

I was hoping you would say that, Dr. McBarbie says. *We will get all the details worked out with insurance, get you on medical leave, and...*

I stand up.

Where are you going?

I thought we were done.

She's worried about me. I can tell, but I just want to go.

Yes, we technically are, but...are you alone in Seattle tonight?

Great. She thinks I'm suicidal. This time, I am not.

Yes, but I'm fine. I swear. I'm just hungry.

I don't sit back down.

I...I knew this would be the outcome. My hand felt just like my right leg felt four years ago, when all of this started. This MRI was a confirmation of what I knew. I just want to get moving on taking care of things before they get worse. I pause but remain standing. *What if the chemo doesn't work?*

Oh, we don't just throw in the towel! We have other options.

Feeling satisfied, I move toward the door.

Suzanne, wait. I am worried about your apparent strength right now. This isn't normal.

I'm mostly just hungry, I tell her and smile.

Ah, the good ol' Suzanne Smile. My neighbor Glenda calls it *dazzling.* I try not to use it as a manipulation technique, but I really need out of here right now. My smile can convince people of anything.

Okay, well, go order some good Seattle food and call me if you need me. Please.

I can't imagine what her life must be like, delivering this news to people all day.

* * *

I try not to bug Jeramy at work, but I call him outside of the hospital.

He answers after the first ring.

Hey, Wiggles.

It's backkkkkk, I say, trying to be funny, and then he lets me cry on the phone for twenty minutes while the sorority girls bitch about their burned chicken nuggets.

I love him.

* * *

I had a ticket to go up in the Space Needle after my appointment, and despite the bad news, it's a sunny Seattle day and I decide to go anyway.

Look at the people having fun!

Look at the tent colonies all over the city!

Look at the one that's on fire!

Look at the girl eating fried tofu in her hotel room after she caught her girlfriend cheating!

Look at the lady in the Space Needle, smiling and taking selfies after hearing her terminal brain cancer has returned!

Pullman, Washington

As I've discovered, there are competitive tiers to chemotherapy.

If you're just taking a pill, then you're lucky. It's not so bad. You shouldn't complain.

Unless you have a port with an IV, you aren't really getting chemo.

That's what some people think.

I get it. I'm glad I don't have an IV or a port, but I'm also here to tell you that port or pill, you feel the shitty side effects all the same.

Lomustine, or as I call it *The Musty*, comes in three pills I swallow at the same time. The sickness comes in dark waves; I feel fine for three hours, and then a murky fog washes over me.

I am fatigued headached nauseated lost broken pained.

The last time I went through this, I couldn't move, but I didn't feel much of anything. I was a sitting tree trunk with everything waving around me, but I felt nothing. This time, I have raging nerve pain in my left hand. I've had this ache before, but nothing showed up on the MRIs, and I brushed the uncomfortable feeling off as nonsense, nothing, anxiety.

I was unfortunately right all along.

I knew this would happen.

Pullman, Washington

My closest friends in Pullman work at the phlebotomy lab.

I know no one here.

At times, I find this isolation appealing. If no one knows me, then no one knows I have cancer. I don't have to explain myself or answer any questions. Sure, I know people ask because they care, but I enjoy the freedom of taking long walks down the college streets, and no one asking about my wonky gait. In the Pacific Northwest, everyone just goes about their business and doesn't study anyone else too closely.[4]

I see my phlebotomy friends once a week. My doctor ordains this, and I can do nothing to stop Dr. McBarbie. My white blood cells vary wildly week-to-week, but other than that, I am fine.

Well, my glucose is always out of range, but of course it is.

Phlebotomist Dustin targets my vein like a hitman whenever I'm assigned to him; he stabs with such accuracy, I want to drag him to Seattle with me when I need MRIs. It's only people like this who can get my veins; former heroin addicts[5] and those who have no fear.

Dustin has no fear.

I don't know what has given him such bravery, but he feels for my vein once and attacks. He doesn't speak to me or tell me stories like the other phlebotomists do. So far, he has my attention.

The woman who works alongside Dustin always has kind words and manifestations for me, but she misses my veins constantly. She tells me about her kid's Halloween costumes, her upcoming engagement *to the man of her freaking dreams*, and how she has *two happy places in her head, the beach in the day and the beach at night*.

I speak back, but I just want her to grow some fangs, sink them deep into my arm, and get me the fuck out of here.

See you next week at 9!

I don't even need to make an appointment.

See?

Friends.

When I call one day because I need to reschedule, a lady answers the phone and says, *Oh my god, Susan, is that you?*

Yep, it's Suzanne! I say.

I totally recognized your voice. You're here so often!

Close enough.

Friends.

Pullman, Washington

On the release day of my new book, I start my second cycle of chemo.

I want to be excited.

This is, after all, quite a thrill.

I never thought I would survive the publication of my first book and certainly not my second.

I already feel horrible, though, and the day won't end well; I'm not a fortune teller or psychic, but I've been through these enough times to know where I'm headed for the week.

Cyclic vomiting. Exhaustion. Never-ending nausea, even if the vomiting isn't so bad.

Today, though I should be celebratory, I'm really fucking tired.

Jeramy texts me: *Be home late from work tonight. Two people got fired!*

Though I know he can't help it, I don't understand why his work crises always seem to happen when I need him here. It's not like I've ever required him to stay home from work or even asked him to leave when I've fallen or been sick. I'm a Low-Maintenance Cancer Patient and have traveled and done everything myself, save for two trips to the local bloodwork center.

Everything.

He's mentioned *my boss told me if I ever need time off, I can have it. If you ever need anything.*

So, no, I'm not happy when he informs me how he will be coming home late on the one night I need him because there is work drama.

But I do my best to deal. I understand he can't sit at home and wait for me to have a cancer crisis that upends his work crisis.

He does the best he can.

I know this.

I just wish I didn't feel so alone.

For so long, I've done most of this by myself, and sometimes, I don't even know how to ask for help. I give the appearance I do—I'll go on social media and request DoorDash gift cards or, in the beginning when I was under the impression people actually wanted to help, asked for rides to radiation, but I shut that down quickly when people actually pushed back.

Now I find it difficult to ask for the smallest things sometimes.

Pullman, Washington

The hospital schedules my next MRI the day before my birthday, and this sends me into such a panic I have to start drinking. Because *everything last time* happened three days after my birthday, I know this has to be a bad sign; nothing about this can be good. This MRI will show if the chemo has been working, but even if it has been, what will happen next?

I have no idea.

I know I'm going on medical leave next semester.

I'm not the online teacher I once was. I'm not the person I once was. I'm not anything I once was.

When thoroughly buzzed, I get a call from a spam number. Before I left Harrisville, I played a free online Bingo game, and if you gave them your phone number, you earned 1,000 free coins. I quit playing the game a week later, but the bastards sold my number and still bother me today.

The number is from Point Pleasant, WV.

278

Home of The Mothman.

I actually answer.

Unless you are The Mothman, I do not want to speak to you.

I take another chug of root beer whiskey straight out of the bottle; I'm alone here, as I am most of the time. No one will notice me or how fast the whiskey disappears.

I had a panic attack in the car earlier over Jeramy drinking coffee with the traveling chef at work because this is absolute bullshit. She keeps asking him to hang out with her, and he keeps lying about it to save face. I can tell he's lying because her messages keep popping up in Microsoft Teams on the shared computer monitor, we use as a television screen.

This morning, he snapped at me before leaving early to hang out with her. Five minutes later, I see he's sent her a message letting her know he's on campus and *has her coffee.*

They are flirting heavily, and I don't appreciate it.

Before he yelled at me for no reason, he told me he had to leave early to *put away a produce truck.* He thinks lying is the way to go, and I also don't appreciate that.

I don't know why he thinks I'm not going to notice he keeps buying or making her coffee every day, especially after he let her borrow a fishing pole.

Oh, and then she asked him to go on a day-long fishing excursion with her, and he told her *he had to think about it.*

He came home and asked me, and I told him there should be no *thinking about it.* There should have been a distinctive *No, that's inappropriate. I have a girlfriend*, but that's not what he said or did. Instead, he seriously told her he *had to think about it.*

I am appalled.

I ask him what he would think if I just met a guy and the guy asked me to go out all day with him fishing while he sat at home with brain cancer.

279

I don't think I would like that too much, he says. *I'll text her and say I can't go.*

I would prefer if you would have said it was inappropriate when she asked you the first time, I say. *I feel disrespected.*

The traveling chefs write a report about us before they go back home, he tells me. *I always want them to say good things about me.* Instead of telling her it's inappropriate because he has a girlfriend, he fucking tells her, *My girlfriend is sick.*

He does this all the time to get out of shit.

I'm tired of being the token sick girlfriend.

All he had to do was say he had a girlfriend.

Not a *sick girlfriend.*

Jeramy frequently says he's *not good with words,* and I understand. Well, I don't understand how he's not good with words, but I understand how I can't follow a recipe and he's an amazing chef, so I try to look at it that way.

But still.

Shot shot shot shot shot shot!

I'm getting progressively drunker as I write this, but so many writers are drunks, the good ones anyway, and most people in my dad's family are drunks, no matter what they tell you, and most of them are liars, but in a funny way, largely, so I do not feel guilty about this.

I am tired of feeling guilty about anything.

I am tired of feeling like I'm not good enough.

I am tired of feeling like I'm going to lose Jeramy whenever he leaves the house *to put away a produce truck* because my brain cancer is back, and there are so many better options out there for him.

I am just tired.

Although I am ill, I clean up after both of us and the pets. I don't cook, but he brings home plenty of food left over from his job. I don't require any of his money; I have my own. I do everything for myself. Whereas most cancer patients with significant others have their people help make appointments, drive them places, navigate insurance policies, and pay for expenses, I don't have him do any of that.

He drove me ten minutes to get bloodwork twice.

It's not that he hasn't offered; I just prefer to do it myself so I don't feel like I owe anyone anything.

However, I think he should realize how lucky he has it. Instead, he snaps at me in the morning, then rushes off to work to have a coffee date with the traveling chef before the day gets started.

I scroll through their other messages. If he's going to have this app on the shared computer on the giant shared television screen, Jeramy should really be more careful.

Traveling Chef: *Can I come over and get some ice for my drink? I got Starbuckies this morning because I'm a basic bitch!*

Smirky face.

Okay, don't tell me you don't have ice in your own kitchen? I'm so over this.

A tray of hotdogs with eight explosion symbols.

Traveling Chef: *Looky what I'm making today.*

Jeramy: *Killin' it.*

Later when we order DoorDash, I snoop through Jeramy's texts. Seems he likes flirting with her on there, too.

Traveling Chef: *Loved what you made earlier. Three stars.*

Jeramy: *Only three?*

Traveling Chef: ;)

Traveling Chef: *Sends ten unnecessary pictures of her cats, mushrooms she found in the wild (Jeramy loves mushroom hunting), her rental truck she named Snowflake (he loves the name, he tells her, and I know why she sends him this: He's been talking about wanting a truck lately to me, and apparently her as well, and romantic pictures of sunsets from her latest trip to Hawaii) *

Jeramy: *Those are awesome!*

Jeramy: *Your lemon bars are...addictive.*

Traveling Chef: *Straight outta the box...* ☺

I'm crushed.

There's a sexual undertone to these texts I can't handle. Sure, he hasn't *done* anything, but this is basically the beginning to an emotional affair, and I'm not having it. Saying her *lemon bars are dot dot dot addictive* is basically the same as saying *hey girl you're addictive, and if I could taste your pussy, it would *also* be addictive.* I don't talk this way to anyone but him, male or female. He doesn't even flirt like this with me through text messages.

If his texts to her sound like this, I hate to think what he says to her in person.

I know the Traveling Chef's type. She's an indie **pick me girl, n.: a girl who befriends men by claiming all the same interests and professing *she's not like other women*.** She now knows Jeramy has a girlfriend, because he did at least tell her that, yet she continues to do this shit because *she's different.* She chooses a rental truck instead of a boring old rental car. She goes morel mushroom hunting instead of exercising at the hotel gym. She plays music *no one has ever heard of* at work, which makes her food somehow taste differently than the other chefs. Her lemon bars *straight outta the box* HAVE SO MUCH MORE FLAVOR than other people's pastries who spend all day working on them. She's just different and cool and more fun than what he has at home, which is a cancerous good for nothing.

It's fine, Jeramy. You can flirt it up with this indie pick me girl at work while I sit in our shitty apartment complex and die of cancer. Hope you're having fun. Hope you're having a fantastic time. Hope she writes an awesome report about sucking your dick.

Shot shot shot shot shot shot!

I decide to call my parents, because ultimately, I want to blame them for having me in the first place, but I need to collapse onto the floor first. It's not a fall. Just a slow decline, symbolic of my cancer journey.

Are you drunk? my mom asks when she finally picks up the phone on my third call.

No, of course not! I say with sudden clarity.

I silently vomit all over the phone, the floor, and my hair.

The chemo is making me sick, I lie. *I need to go.*

I'm pissed at Jeramy, but I don't want him to come home to whiskey vomit all over the floor. I am not great, but I am better than this. I wipe everything up the best I can and throw myself in the shower.

I know the Traveling Chef has asked him to do other things and he's lied because he's a horrible liar.

Finally, he comes clean. *Yeah, she asked both of us to go bowling, and I said no.*

Why did you do that? I might have actually given her a bit more credit if I would have known she also asked me to do something.

He didn't even mention this to me, but I knew something had gone down.

Can you imagine you trying to bowl? You can't even stand up.

Killin' it, I think. *Winky fucking face.*

Pullman, Washington

My third round of chemo leaves me devastatingly-cry-in-the-shower-sick. I can't move without vomiting or feeling like my head is going to fall off my body. When Jeramy leaves for work, I turn off every light and try to sleep for a few more hours.

Sometimes it works, sometimes it doesn't.

On the weekend, he makes a fuss about lighting candles and incense all over the apartment because he *can't stand the smell of puke.* I've flushed and wiped everything down and seriously can't take a weird accusation like this.

You should be kinder with your words, I tell him. *It's not my fault I have cancer and am puking.*

Yeah, you're right, he says, but then he just goes on like nothing is wrong. *I'm sorry,* he says, but I don't believe him. I can barely move or walk or function, and he's just sitting in the living room playing a video game.

For hours.

I get that he has worked all week, but I need him to pay attention to me. I've been alone and vomiting, and this? Sitting in front of a video game all weekend? I've seen the way significant others who care about sick loved one's act, and this ain't it.

We've been through this before.

Well, just tell me what you need, and I'll do it.

I kinda feel like we are past that, though. It should just be intuitive at this point. You should know what I need when I don't feel well.

I'm not going to bring a person water who isn't thirsty.

I wonder what's wrong with him.

We've been together a year, and he struggles to say he cares about me.

Quite frequently, I ask myself why I'm here. Why I love him so much. Why I knock myself out to clean the apartment and provide him with everything he needs and wants when he barely notices me.

Jeramy and I watch paranormal videos[6] all the time, and I already feel like a ghost in his life.

When I confront him about this, he swears it isn't true. He does care about me. He just *doesn't know how to act or what to do.*

None of this is easy; I have to know this by now.

I try to understand, but when on the sickest day I've ever had he looks me straight in the eye and says he's *going to go throw some discs,* I don't fucking understand.

I don't fucking understand at all.

I want to tell him that as a partner of someone with active brain cancer, he does not have the right to go *throw some discs* on my sickest day.

I feel guilty about this.

Perhaps I am asking too much.

I always am.

Nowhere

Why is she even on chemo? the doctor says. I have never seen this doctor. I don't know him, but he's clearly been assigned to me through some unfortunate stroke of horrible luck. *Chemo isn't going to save her. Her brain's too far gone. I don't know why we are bothering with this.*

I am dreaming. I can't control anything, so I'm terrified. I've never seen this doctor before, and he's discussing me like I'm not even in the room.

I try to speak but can't.

I hate when I dream about brain cancer.

Sleep is my only respite; brain cancer patients love sleep. (Often, we also have insomnia, which is one of the great oxymorons of brain tumors.)

But this doctor keeps screaming at me; he won't leave me

be. I'm in his office, but something feels off. It's dirty, like a makeshift medical room in a foreign country, and there are off-white sheets hanging to separate my section from other patients. Everyone can hear this doctor yelling about *how we have wasted our significant cancer resources on this woman who is obviously going to die.* I can feel the red rising up through my olive skin.

This isn't embarrassment, though.

This is shame.

I have wasted resources that could have saved someone else.

In the dream, I remember when I was first diagnosed and told I qualified for a clinical trial. Believing I would never last a few months, I thought the clinical trial would be beneficial for others who suffered from glioblastoma, which was my diagnosis at the time. I took the high road and thought I was doing *something good.* If I couldn't survive, hopefully I could help others.

I believed this.

Then my doctor looked at me and said, *No, this is to help you.*

I was taken aback.

I had already given up hope; not in a negative way, but in a *this is just how it is: my reality* sort of way.

Then the guy in the clinical trial, a few pills ahead of me, croaked or nearly croaked and the whole thing was called off, but anyway.

Get this woman out of here! She is just using us! We shouldn't have her in here. This is ridiculous.

The doctor throws clipboards. He refuses to make eye contact with me. He has more than one vein bulging in his forehead, which I didn't know was possible.

I suddenly realize I recognize my doctor. It's Coach Steve from the North Carolina hotel room that smelled of bus seats.

I have never had an oncologist like this in my waking life. They've been good, kind people. They've given everything they can to me.

This woman does not fucking deserve our resources!

A flurry of loose-leaf papers flies toward me like birds with sharp wings, and a few cut my face. I touch my skin and feel blood, as if the shame has hemorrhaged from my cheeks. My story leaks onto the pages before fluttering away.

I...I didn't mean to. I want to leave.

No one pays attention to me. It's like I'm not here.

I squeeze my eyes shut in the dream and am engulfed by darkness. I hear the dripping water and know where I am.

Never has this been about me.

Not then, when I had my initial seizure.

Not when I had brain surgery.

Not when I relearned to walk.

Not when I did radiation or chemo.

Not when I persevered and beat every damn cancerous cell in my brain.

Not when I survived two different types of abusive relationships.

Not when I moved home to help my parents.

Not when I trekked across the country with a new love.

Not when my cancer came back.

But when I was walking through those tunnels, falling, and digging through the mud to get back up?

That was about me.

That's when I found myself.

As the crazed doctor's screams fade into the darkness and drift away from me, I smile.

I am in control now.

. . .

Nowhere

Text to Emily: You just got a bunch of weird sex poems for *Dead Skunk* in the email today. The guy sent fifteen.

Text back from Emily: *completely glossing over the weird sex part because we get inappropriate shit all the time* He sent fifteen? The guidelines clearly say only send three. Ugh.

Pullman, Washington

Nurse Bianca calls on Thanksgiving Eve with bad news.

Jeramy prepares Thanksgiving dinner in our miniscule apartment kitchen. I told him he didn't have to do anything, but he tells me cooking will be relaxing for him.

We are *working on things.* I know dating someone with a terminal illness can't be easy, so I forgive him. He forgives me for screaming at him about his emotional affair. Sometimes I fear he doesn't want to be with me because *things have changed*, but we move forward into the dark uneasiness.

My bloodwork *looks great!* Nurse Bianca tells me with enthusiasm.

This is not the bad news.

Nurse Bianca is so nice and always cheerful; I don't know how she stays this way. Her job has got to be extremely difficult, but she's one of those people who always sounds like she's smiling when she speaks. Did she work in customer service before she became a brain tumor nurse? Or is she really just that accommodating?

Maybe both.

Who knows, but the Alvord Brain Tumor Center is lucky to have Nurse Bianca.

The bad news.

We're shipping your chemo to you tomorrow, and you can begin as soon as you get it.

Wait.

I act as if I knew this was coming, but I didn't. I thought I would only start chemo again after my next MRI, which is the day before my birthday. I thought I was getting a break. I thought I was getting a little time off.

Okay, great! I say with a smile.

I, too, once worked in customer service.

I think you said you needed to get some dental work done? Nurse Bianca asks. It's true—since radiation, I've needed a shit ton of dental work. Something about sending high-energy rays into my face and head seemed to do a lot of damage to my mouth, and it's cost me thousands of dollars since then.

Oh, the aftereffects of cancer no one discusses.

You survived but you will pay—lots of money and great parts of your sanity—for remaining amongst the living.

Um, yes, I need a crown—a crown put on.

Jeramy stops messing with the turkey he's brining. I guess I also have Resting Can't Fucking Hide Anything Voice, and he can tell I'm agitated.

Okay, well, usually we want you to start the chemo right away.

I really need to get this tooth taken care of.

I don't tell this to Nurse Bianca, but somedays, I feel like my smile is the one physical piece of me I have left. I've lost weight, I've gained weight, I've lost weight and kept it off this time, I've looked as dead as a tunnel ghost behind my brown eyes, but my smile has been the one thing I remember about myself when I look into the mirror. I don't want to ruin any of my teeth.

I need this dental work done, chemo be damned.

Do you promise to start the chemo right after your dental work?

Of course!

Both of our customer service voices have returned; Nurse Bianca and I understand one another.

When I get off the phone, I'm a little shaken. I try to play it off—after all, tomorrow is Thanksgiving and Jeramy's birthday. I want the day to be about him and not me, for once. Too much of this relationship, our relationship, is not about me, but my cancer. He deals with this well, too well sometimes, it makes me worry about his mental health. These coming days should be about him.

You're already starting chemo again? he says, holding turkey legs like a deer he's just shot in the woods.

I guess so, I say, trying to smile. *I...thought I would get a break.*

I forgot: Cancer doesn't take breaks.

Oh, I'm sorry, he says as he contorts the turkey's legs as if the bird is a circus acrobat.

Relaxing, he says.

I don't say anything. What is there to say?

* * *

Later, I help him roll dough. My fine motor skills still blow, but it's fun.

You would never guess Jeramy is a fantastic baker—his wooly beard and calloused hands make him seem like more of a butcher, as his grandfather was. The juxtaposition is one of the quirks I like about him so much. His breads, cookies, and desserts are the best I've ever had. He calls baking *his curse*—he hates nothing more than whipping up *the best batch of pumpkin spice cupcakes this sorority has ever had!* but it's what he does best.

But bread.

He likes baking bread.

290

Dough is forgiving, he tells me as we make little circles with the mixture. *You can't mess it up.*

I think about how demanding and unforgiving all my past relationships have been. As we let the dough rest, I am thankful that like the bread, this relationship is the most forgiving.

Nowhere

Although cancer eats my brain faster than the ghost, I saw floating through Tunnel #17, my thoughts are quicker.

I often imagine what kind of woman Jeramy will be with after me.

I have this odd feeling he will have a couple one-night stands and feel strange about it later, maybe even a bit guilty, before taking an extended vacation to Thailand for a few months, or maybe Alaska, and then upon return, realize the stable woman from work he asked to watch our cats is actually pretty cute and maybe he would like to take her out for sushi as a thank you. She just got out of a long-term relationship a few months ago, so she's not really ready for anything either, but they enjoy each other's company and friendship.

The *sushi thank you thing* isn't really a date, but he pays for it and can't help but think about how we came to the same spot our second night in town, and the server yelled at the business men beside us because they wouldn't leave her alone, how it was between casual flirting for a bigger tip and being actually annoyed with them, *you can see I am really busy here, but you won't leave me alone now, will you?*, and how either way, the men would not take the hint, and we felt sorry for her and found her unrequited banter hilarious. *Oops I might accidentally drop a sea creature pancake on your lap if you bug me again, Mr. Businessman!* and we were openly laughing at all of it.

Then he will drive home the girl who watched our cats, and she will be kind of hopeful, because although she isn't quite over her ex-boyfriend, she wouldn't mind ending the night with a nice kiss or two, and that's a lot to wish for, but her co-worker with the cats is so mysterious with those pale blue eyes, and though she's relatively certain he doesn't have a girlfriend, he's definitely never mentioned one, she does find a purple hairclip in the armrest of the passenger seat, and she absentmindedly clicks it open and shut as he tells her about this fish he caught in Alaska. Maybe the hairclip belonged to a sister or niece or something, though he hasn't mentioned either of those, not yet. It most definitely belonged to an ex, or maybe a current girl? Maybe the *sushi thank you thing* really was just a thank you and nothing more, and they would just see each other at work the next day like they didn't have fish, rice, and good conversation the evening before.

Hey, thanks for coming out with me this evening, he tells her. *I had a nice time. You're good company.*

And she doesn't know this, but he's feeling guilty, like I'm waiting at home for him, mad he took another woman on a date. He knows I would find this inappropriate if I were alive, and I would cry if I knew he took another woman out for sushi and regaled her with stories about all the big fish he caught in Alaska.

She doesn't know he only really likes to talk on car rides, and her apartment is a good ten miles from the sushi restaurant.

She also doesn't know *good company* is his code for *I like you.*

Yeah, you, too! she replies, a little too enthusiastically.

Clip. Unclip. Clip. Unclip.

We could maybe do it again sometime, he says with his eyes on the road. Unlike me, Jeramy is a safe driver.

But this girl is a thinker, just like I was, and she can sense something is strange. Girls don't leave random hairclips in cars unless they are in that vehicle a lot. It's not like an important ring or necklace they "forget" over at an apartment as a manipulative scheme to see a guy again; an easily replaceable hairclip is something that just gets left behind, like a spare sock. Something no one has to think about, an item that is just there when you need it.

This was serious.

Clip. Unclip. Clip. Clip.

Something with Hairclip Girl went down, and it went down hard. Sure, she probably thinks it was a rough breakup. Sure, she has no idea he took care of me when I had a brain cancer recurrence.

Sure, she doesn't know the hairclip belongs to his dead girlfriend, and he just hasn't noticed it's still in the car.

Sure, she hasn't been inside his apartment yet, our apartment, to see the pictures of us still on the wall.

Sure, she hasn't been around him outside of work long enough for him to open up and say, *So I was with this girl for a long time, and she died.*

Suzanne.

Clip. Unclip. Was this thing broken? Clip.

Yeah...we could do this again. It's just...work, it might be weird, she says.

Oh, I mean, yeah, no big deal, just friends, you know.

Yeah, of course, she says, a bit disappointed. She hoped he would bring up his past a bit, maybe say, *so there was this bad breakup I had, this girl I had a little trouble getting over,* and then they could bond over their horrible exes and maybe, she doesn't know, casually fuck or something, suck the sadness right out of their fortysomething bodies so she doesn't have to get on the lonely dating apps later, but he jumped to *just being friends,* and somehow I would sit in the backseat, a ghost from all the paranormal videos he and I once watched, and flick that hairclip right out of her tiny pale hands toward the windshield.

Whoa, whoa, he says. *No need to get upset,* and then he would grab her hand and make her more confused than ever.

Jeramy tells me when I die, it *will hurt for a long time, but then he will move on.* I don't know why he thinks he should tell me this, and I get pissed off. I don't want to hear this. Of course, he's going to move on. Who wouldn't? But why does he feel the need to say this aloud, especially when I'm in pain? I don't understand.

I don't think he means to hurt me, but I sink deeper and deeper into the bed, our bed, a bed he will probably get rid of once I die because it will feel weird to sleep in once I'm gone, and I sink into it until I disappear like that forgotten hairclip his new friend will find in his car, and soon enough, no one will know I was there at all.

Pullman, Washington

The tech does not make me take off any of my clothes for the MRI.

He also does not make me remove my boots.

He does not insert an IV.

I start panicking.

One question, I say. *When do we do the whole IV thing?*

Oh, we do things a little differently here. We just spent a ton of money upgrading our equipment, so we insert the IV later.

As someone who has had a lot of MRIs, this makes zero sense to me. The IV always goes in before the scan begins; even if they don't administer the gadolinium until halfway through the scan, most techs want the IV first.

This is weird.

Pullman is not Seattle. I am not sure I should trust this process, no matter how much money they just spent.

Okay.

And into the tube I go.

I am worried this isn't going to work. Dr. McBarbie, who is on top of everything, is going to call the next day and tell me I need to redo everything. Am I going to have to pay for two scans? I'm not going to be able to do that. It's right before Christmas, for crying out loud. And I need these results. I need to know if I'm going to require surgery, radiation, *the works.*

Halfway through the scan, my new friend comes back, and I think it's to administer an IV. This should be easier than last time. At least my veins should be popping from that warm blanket. I'm also flat on my back and can't see shit and for me, this is probably a good thing.

You're going back in! the tech says gleefully.

Wait a minute. I felt nothing. Assuming there's a line in my arm, I stay corpse still. I anticipate the cold shock and bitter taste of the chemical in my mouth, but nothing happens. Before I know it, I'm out of the tube, and the tech helps me down from the table.

There is no cord in my arm or anywhere near it.

All I have is a bandage.

I sit there a moment and try to figure out what happened.

Are you feeling okay? the tech asks. He genuinely seems to care.

Yeah...I'm just a little confused.

Seems like they are just monitoring you for maintenance this time. Don't worry! I followed all the orders.

It just...seemed too easy.

I guess I have MRI trauma from the one scan where the IV insertion took over five hours and my arm almost blew up. I feel like something should have gone wrong.

So...can I ask what happened to you?

Sometimes people want to know.

I don't mind.

I have boiled three memoirs down to two minutes.

He wishes me a Merry Christmas, and I do the same for him.

Pullman, Washington

I once loved my birthday.

It was one of the most selfish things about me.

Maybe it's a Sagittarius issue; I'm not sure.

Yes, I know, astrology is bullshit, but it's kinda fun sometimes.

Everything happened three days after my birthday four years ago.

Each year, the PTSD softens a bit. The first year after *everything happened*, I spent most of the day in my car screaming in an abandoned parking lot. As cathartic as it was, this might have traumatized me more.

I don't remember what happened the second year.

I seriously have zero memory of it.

The third year, I picked up Olive Garden (Mom) and Outback (Dad) in Parkersburg and did some screaming and crying in my car, but not nearly as much. *I had come so far.* I had improved my walking.

I had found most of the thirteen tunnels by that point.

I had even managed to get into what I imagined would be a healthy relationship.

But still, I needed to scream.

This year, I have a stomach virus and am on chemo.

Is it a virus or my body saying *nah, you know what this is. This is me reminding you of the trauma you experienced four years ago. This is your body telling you that you'll never be the fucking same. You know exactly what's happening here.*

I vomit I vomit I vomit.

I have a telehealth appointment with Dr. McBarbie on December 21st.

No one needs to remind me: That was my surgery day four years ago.

Please tell me I don't need another surgery please tell me I don't need another surgery please tell me I don't need another surgery.

I have to wait and see.

Pullman, Washington

December 18, otherwise known as *The Day Everything Happened*, arrives without fanfare. It's a day just like any other day for most people, but for me, it's a PTSD fiery hell. I'm in my head from the minute I wake up, and I can't stop thinking something bad will happen to me or someone else I care about.

Four years ago, I sat at a coffee shop with a friend who wouldn't be my friend a few months later, having a seizure I thought was a Charley Horse, thinking maybe I had a stroke and was going to drive six hours home soon.

Instead, my life became a horror show of living in hospitals and hotels, relearning to walk, and surviving from one radiation treatment to the next.

Within seconds, the creature growing in my brain, the thing that didn't belong, decided to make itself known and wreak havoc, causing me to lose control of the right side of my body and rely on mobility aids and luck to transport myself from one step to the next.

I stopped being an English professor, a friend, a roller derby teammate, and a potential romantic partner. The only piece of me that didn't change was the part of me that could write. The writing still existed. Somehow, I was still me.

But now.

Four years later, I feel like that's disappearing.

Words don't look the same.

They morph into different letters, even numbers, before my eyes. Everything is a kaleidoscope of skunk-colored blended words I can't even distinguish sometimes.

I am dying.

I have thought this before.

I seem fine all day.

Jeramy thinks this until I am rinsing a plate over and over again, although it's been clean for three minutes now. I burst into tears, and he can't figure out what's wrong. I can tell he's uncomfortable, but he tries to fix the problem.

You can't fix the problem, I tell him in my mind. I'm sure he hears me. I just need this hug, and I don't want him to let me go.

Why are you crying?

Does he really not know? He doesn't. I remember; he's never been through any life-changing event like this, and for that I am glad.

I told you it would be a hard day.

He remembers.

Right, right, of course. You just seemed fine all day.

I was. It's just...I'm not fine now, though. It's complicated.

You seemed fine.

I'm still crying, and I can't stop. I wasn't really fine all day. I just buried myself in busy work so I wouldn't have to think about this horrible shit. Eventually, though, when I was cleaning an already spotless dish, I lost my shit. I couldn't hold it in any longer. I started thinking about everything that happened, little flashes here and there, quick little bursts of light and darkness interspersed with needles, numbness, and no sleep.

I look away for a moment, and when I glance back, Jeramy clasps his hands above his head and gyrates his hips, a special dance he does only for me when I'm sad.

I laugh because what else can I do?

He's a fantastic dancer.

Later, I beg Jeramy to stay awake with me, and he does for as long as he can. We are opposites in a lot of ways, though, and he falls asleep when his head even senses a pillow. I get up to eat some cheese and stand in the living room.

I can't figure out why I'm standing there. I can't move. I'm like a fucking ice sculpture, frozen and then melting very quickly as my seizures begin. Once they start, they don't stop. I have never lost consciousness during my seizures, thankfully, which is the one nice aspect of my brand of brain cancer.

Now I don't dare move.

I'm afraid to.

My seizures emerge from fear.

Scared I'm going to fall?

Seizure.

Scared I'm going to lose my mind?

Seizure.

Scared I'm going to have a terrible MRI result the same day I had a craniotomy four years ago?

Three or four seizures.

There's nothing I can do to stop them.

Jeramy has told me they are scary to watch. I wouldn't know. I just have to let them happen, wait until they are over so I can get on with my day.

Pullman, Washington

I don't want to get out of bed for this telehealth appointment.

I shouldn't complain; all I need to do is walk to the living room.

I am in space.

On the Zoom call I am in space, anyway. This is a leftover background from my book release party, which went well, I think. I did get booted from the party once, accidentally, but after that, everything seemed to go smoothly.

The nurse who liked my snack backpack tells me she wants to refer to me by my title, so she calls me *Doctor Suzanne*. I'm not sure where she's even getting this info (probably somewhere in my patient history?), but I tell her to *please just call me Suzanne*. I don't want my brain cancer nurse, who is honestly way smarter than I am, referring to me as doctor anything.

Suzanne will be just fine.

I oscillate between reallyfuckingnervous and unnaturally-fuckingcalm, and this is what the last four years have turned me into.

Agiganticfuckingmessinsidemyhead.

We will go with that.

The nurse tells me Doctor McBarbie will be late, and I'm cool with that. I sit in the virtual waiting room with Jeramy, who seems way more reallyfuckingnervous than I do. I'm not accustomed to seeing him like this, *nervous*, and this frightens me more than anything.

When Dr. McBarbie arrives, she reads me a disclaimer like a used car salesman. It's a new telehealth requirement, she informs me, and I smile and wait.

I can't change what happens, I remind myself. No matter how long this takes, the result is the same. I don't mind waiting because at the end of the day, I can't alter what the MRI says.

The MRI reads you.

You don't read the MRI.

Dr. McBarbie inquires about my latest seizures, and I tell her about the *twitchy feelings* I have when I'm falling asleep. It feels like I'm sinking into the tunnels I once explored, dark and full of unknowns. The twitching never stops, and because of the fussing, I don't sleep. I wake up every hour or so to readjust, thinking I will feel more comfortable, but I don't.

I just keep falling deeper and deeper into dark unknowns with zero light on the other side.

I'm going to suggest Klonopin for the seizures, she says. *I see you took that once for anxiety; how did it make you feel?*

Um, I am stumped. *Okay, I guess. I didn't feel out of it or anything the next day. I was fine.*

Okay, we are going to try that.

I start spinning a little. Klonopin for seizures? Dr. McBarbie knows way more than I do, but I've never heard of this before. I don't know how this will help. Are my twitching sensations psychological? Yes, some things happened, some very weird things, like dead bugs beginning to move and people appearing who weren't really there at all, but I don't think I'm crazy.

Sounds good! I chirp.

Jeramy clears his throat. He's the type of guy who doesn't even take Tylenol when he has a headache. What's he going to think of someone knocked out on K-pins to stop seizures? At least he has heard the Klonopin is for seizures and not anything else, or he might be done with me forever now. No, I assure myself. He's still just nervous. Dr. McBarbie is doing her small talk dance and hasn't started in with the actual reason for the appointment.

Did you see the good news already? Dr. McBarbie asks.

My brown eyes gleam gold. She said *good news. GOOD NEWS.* I haven't heard these words in so long that I wonder if she somehow shot me up with liquid Klonopin through the computer screen. I am in space, after all.

I am in the center of the universe.

I am flying. I am living. I am alive.

No! No, I have not seen the good news!

I don't think I actually said this aloud.

I am silent.

I thought you might have actually seen the report before I did, she says. *I've been looking forward to this appointment all day.*

No, no I haven't seen anything. Please tell me.

I am! So! Excited!

If I was physically able to stand and dance, I would.

She starts in about how the MRI looks a little strange because it's *sliced differently and shows different planes of my brain* or something like that. To be perfectly honest, I have no idea what she's talking about. I heard *good news* and that's all I need to know.

I am trying to listen for details, but I am too elated.

I feel like I'm flipping through my spirit box and all I'm hearing is *your. scan. looks. great.*

I hear Dr. McBarbie's voice as I drift off to sleep that night.

Everything is going to be fine.

PART VI
THE END

Pullman, Washington

Despite the positive MRI, I begin to sharply decline after the new year. My seizures increase. I stop tolerating the chemo. I can't keep my eyes open because of the headaches. I spend more time puking than awake and alert.

I'm barely functional, and I want this to be over.

The Internet

I search everywhere for people who have HGAP brain tumors.

My search yields nothing.

Where are they?

I can't be the only one, but it seems they aren't looking for me.

One day, some really smart people will discuss HGAP in medical journals, and they will use the *Frontal Matter Trilogy* as an odd source.

I just know it.

I do.

Pullman, Washington

When you have brain cancer, good news never lasts long. I am doing my daily five-mile walk at the local coliseum when the lady who smokes the clove cigarettes and works there stops me and says, *Honey, you don't look so good? Are you okay?*

No, I am not.

She helps me to my car, and I drive back to the apartment and try to convince myself the weakness in my legs is a fluke.

Jeramy rushes home from work early and takes me to the ER, where they do an emergency MRI.

There are not one, but two new tumors on my left side. This is out of control. I will stop my chemo immediately and head to Seattle to be admitted.

Pullman, Washington

I don't make it to Seattle fast enough.

I wake up after the ER and can't feel either of my legs.

I wake up the next morning and can't feel my waist.

This didn't even happen in 2017.

I am scared shitless.

I am totally dependent on Jeramy to lift me on the toilet and into bed.

I don't know what I'd do without him.

I really didn't want it to be like this, but thank the Mothman he's here.

Seattle, Washington

Dr. McBarbie sees me in the pods and levels with me before I am admitted to the hospital.

I am not strong enough for chemo, but I can receive a dosage of intravenous immunotherapy called Avastin beforehand. It's *shown great promise in brain cancer patients*, and what do I have to lose?

Then she discusses hospice. If things don't improve, that's where I'll be. *I'm nervous about both of your stoicism*, she says because she cares.

This isn't stoicism, though.

This is just seeing the future.

* * *

I group text Sarah and Emily because I only have the strength to text it once.

Emily immediately books a flight and will be in Seattle promptly. Sarah? She will be in Pullman soon and has *big plans to redecorate the apartment!*

I don't blame her; it's the only way she knows how to deal.

I am placed on the cardiac unit because there are no rooms on the neurology floor. A nurse immediately removes my catheter from the Pullman ER and tells me I'll *be using a bedpan from here on out.*

I have no idea how humiliating this is going to get.

I will spend the next five nights with my head on a bed towel because it's more comfortable than a pillow.

I will have to watch funny *Family Feud* clips to feel comfortable enough to take a shit in a bedpan, with no real clue if I'm actually aiming correctly or not.

I will spend far too long sitting in my own urine because of *understaffing issues*, and I cry when Emily gets there. She rushes to give me a hug, and I feel heard.

I will have a constant parade of doctors in-and-out of my room to see if the steroids are helping me move (they are, but with the constant threat of dangerously high blood sugars), to see if I can actually get out of bed (I can, to everyone's surprise, especially Dr. McBarbie), and to see if a medication named Baclofen is aiding my night terrors (it is!).

A night nurse named Ami will save my life.

I nominate her for an award.

She deserves so much more than that for wiping my ass every single night.

Pullman, Washington

No one can believe I'm walking again, and to my delight, after a week of resting at home and watching old *Unsolved Mysteries* with Emily (we love the SCI-MED cases but don't know exactly what that means) while Jeramy works, Dr. McBarbie tells me I can try the Carboplatin chemo.

I am thrilled.

I don't know that the first dosage will cause me to lose 23 pounds in two weeks, throw up every sip of water I swallow, and be unable to move from my bed for three weeks.

I am not thrilled.

I am horrified.

I decide to pull the plug on the chemo but continue the immunotherapy.

I don't want my last moments to be full of vomit.

Sarah and Emily's visits intersect for a short time, and I hear them moving an air mattress into the hallway and erupting into fits of giggles as they try to coerce the bed down the narrow path. When I see it stuck the next morning, Emily says, *I wanted to move it into the living room, but Sarah said she liked it there.*

I am eternally grateful.

Pullman, Washington

I know the end is coming soon.

I call my parents crying. My mom says I've *been the joy of her life and am the strongest person* she knows. This means more to me than I tell her.

The seizures keep increasing, which I know isn't a positive sign. One night, my teeth won't stop clacking and grinding; this goes on for hours. I put in an old roller derby mouth guard to ease the pain and briefly remember my old life.

Skating. Lucky. Free.

Another night, I am standing at our counter, and I feel a rubber band snap in my brain. I black out and hit the ground while seizing, which has never happened before.

How long can I survive this?

How?

Who?

I am a writer.

I am a ~~brilliant~~ writer.

I am a writer.

No one will ever take that away from me.

Not a person, not a teacher, not a parent, not a relationship, not cancer.

I was born for this.

I was made to write.

I was made to share what happened to me.

It's always scary, it's always intimidating, and it's always wrong.

This is what makes it so right.

This is what makes it real.

I am nothing more than a big blubbering fish caught on a line at Spring Valley Lake, where Jeramy taught me to cast.

Jeramy is good, the best dancer I know, the person who made the end of my life worth living.

I am sick.

I am full of life and darkness.

I am dying.

I am real.

Sometimes I think cats are the only beings to understand me.

Maybe ghosts.

I am not real, I am sure of this.

I never make sense to myself.

Time doesn't seem real when you have brain cancer.

People think I am mean, but mostly, I am just realistic. I don't cut the corners of emotions. I feel anything and everything. I feel what I feel. I feel what you feel. I feel what they feel. I feel what you don't want to feel. I understand what you're going through, or at least I will try to. I will give you the ultimate benefit of the doubt until I am crushed.

I love you I love you I love you.

I fall in love with all the people who don't love me back, and that's okay.

I am always a little behind the curve.

Sometimes I feel too much, and I like to feel too much. I will always love you, like Dolly, not like Whitney because she was a little too rock-and-roll, and I'm always a little bit country.

Some people never text me back, and I care. I care about that a lot.

I've had very few sexual partners, and sometimes, that bothers me.

I am very sad most of the time because I love my life, and now it's over.

I don't know how long I've had brain tumors but apparently, it's been longer than most people have known.

I've had amazing moments on the dance floor.

I am, for the most part, a very structured person.

I often hide behind my smile.

I am 100% a cat person who also loves dogs.

I feel strange if I don't write every single day.

I know the end is coming soon.

The MRIs with the tumors growing everywhere in my brain have provided a map to death, have shown me just how much time I have left. The glowing masses keep getting bigger and bigger and bigger and I know Dr. McBarbie will eventually say, *Look, Suzanne, I'm sorry—there's nothing we can do but keep you comfortable* because Dr. McBarbie is a practical person, which I love and need.

Everyone says they don't know what happens when they die, but I know, oh I know exactly the way this will go: I will head down that dark tunnel, my favorite, #12, and it will be black upon entry because I am leaving this world, and I am frightened there will be nothing but emptiness to look forward to forever. I will walk alone and fear falling, as I have always done, but I will keep pushing forward and moving and wondering what comes next, even if it's vacuous space.

This is just who I am.

And then suddenly, as if my subconscious creates my surroundings, a pinprick of light will appear before me and get wider and brighter as I keep moving forward. My legs, once useless under me, will feel weightless and free as I run toward the dazzling opening at the other end of #12. Although the tunnel is rife with mud and water, I will not get stuck or fall as I once did.

As if I am abandoning winter for spring, the opening of the

tunnel will illuminate before me, and I will realize I'm not walking at all but being carried.

I was waiting for you, he will whisper.

Bright red eyes will blink at me like a cat and furry wings will wrap around my torso to keep me safe.

I am leaving this life.

I will not come back to these hills, valleys, mountains, or deserts.

I will not come back to these heartbreaks.

The Mothman will carry me home under his giant black wings, and I will finally be safe forever.

THE AFTER

Outside of Seattle, Snoqualmie Tunnel, Snoqualmie pass, 11,894 ft.

I look at Jeramy and flip on my headlamp.

This tunnel is over two-and-a-half miles long. Think you can handle it? There's a waterfall at the end.

Jeramy clasps his hands above his head and gyrates his hips, a special dance he does only for me. I laugh.

Ready, Wiggles.

We head into the deep darkness, unafraid of what we cannot see.

ACKNOWLEDGMENTS

Thank you to Amanda D'Agostino for the gorgeous paintings; Barbara for her patient editing; Lisa for willingness to let me try new ideas; Emily for her dedication to SCI-MED and *Dead Skunk*; Sarah for YUPPPP!; my parents for not reading a word of these books; Loren, Kyle, Kelly, Meg, William, and Cathleen for rabbit rabbit; Amanda for always backing me up; Vanessa, Jessica, Jodi, Travis, Waggle, Nodya, Carrie, Neecee, Shelley, Amy, Betsy, Ninja, Wrex, Lisa S., Rolli, Josh S., and Jesse for years of friendship; Cole, Kate, Gail, and Peaches for keeping me sane; "Tuckie" for being my writing mentor; and, of course, Jeramy for making all of this worth it.

IN MEMORIUM

On September 17, 2022, the literary world, indeed the whole world, lost a unique voice with the passing of Suzanne "Hammer" Samples. Her final journey began in 2014 with a brain tumor diagnosis. She chronicled her struggles and triumphs even as she worked through post-surgery rehab including regaining the loss of arm and hand function. Suzanne's rare courage and candor gave us a brutally honest and unflinching view of her life. Though she "nagged" her editor and publisher to get her first book into print before she died, Suzanne outlived her prognosis. The memoir, "Frontal Matter: Glue Gone Wild" went on to be named among the best books of 2019 by Kirkus Reviews and sent Suzanne on a phenomenal book tour where she wowed listeners with her experiences, stellar personality and dark wit. She continued on to write two sequels, "Stargazing in Solitude" published to acclaim in 2021, and the "13 Tunnels", even as she returned to teaching and started a literary magazine. Her trilogy offers insight, comfort, and understanding to the patients, caregivers, and loved ones

319

dealing with this and similar devastating diagnoses. Suzanne lived life to the fullest and gave us great gifts along the way. She will be missed.

-- Barbara Lockwood and Lisa Kastner

Running Wild Press publishes stories that cross genres with great stories and writing. RIZE publishes great genre stories written by people of color and by authors who identify with other marginalized groups. Our team consists of:

Lisa Diane Kastner, Founder and Executive Editor
Mona Bethke, Acquisitions Editor, RIZE
Benjamin White, Acquisition Editor, Running Wild
Peter A. Wright, Acquisition Editor, Running Wild
Resa Alboher, Editor
Rebecca Dimyan, Editor
Andrew DiPrinzio, Editor
Abigail Efird, Editor
Henry L. Herz, Editor
Laura Huie, Editor
Cecilia Kennedy, Editor
Barbara Lockwood, Editor
Kelly Powers, Reader
Cody Sisco, Editor
Chih Wang, Editor
Pulp Art Studios, Cover Design
Standout Books, Interior Design
Polgarus Studios, Interior Design

Learn more about us and our stories at www.runningwild-press.com

Loved this story and want more? Follow us at www.run-ningwildpress.com, www.facebook/runningwildpress, on Twitter @lisadkastner @RunWildBooks

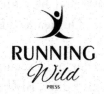

NOTES

EPIGRAPH

1. I took these notes from my prolific uncle's work titled *ALL ABOUT THE CLAN*. Though named Mack, my father often refers to his brother as "The Mackaroon," and for reasons I don't quite understand, "The Godfather."

1. This was reported in the *Point Pleasant Register*, Point Pleasant, WV Wednesday, on November 16, 1966. I'm not going to give an MLA citation because honestly, as someone who has been teaching for over a decade, I'm tired of proper citations. This is a CREATIVE ENDEAVOR.
2. App-uh-latch-uns for this area, please. Otherwise, I'll throw an apple atcha.
3. Indrid Cold, or The Smiling Man, is typically associated with UFO activity and *might* be an alien or *perhaps* in cahoots with The Men in Black. He quite often showed up around the same areas and similar times as The Mothman, hence the association.

1. My mom also believed I had a sinus infection when I had a brain tumor, so I guess that is her go to?
2. This might seem like a strange thing to include, but a weird boy I knew showed me a dolphin porn video after school one day, and I've never been able to shake the image from my understanding of the internet's infancy.
3. Apparently, those are a thing.
4. He did not kill Osama Bin Laden, though he claimed to multiple times.
5. To an extent. Anyone who blabbers on and on about an ex probably isn't over them and might need to do some serious self-reflection.
6. I find this odd because I've obviously dated both men and women. I guess he doesn't feel threatened by women. Who would know?
7. The Fogwoman: Alaskan god-like creature from *Stargazing in Solitude*.
8. The unofficial food of West Virginia, the pepperoni roll was originally created as a quick lunch for coal miners. Now, it's an Appalachian

delicacy.

9. I despise the word *supper*. I don't really have a reason; I much prefer *dinner*.

10. After I eschewed the weird Optune space helmet that required I keep my head shaved, my hair started to grow back. We all know this is a *sign of health*. I've also faced the reality I have become obese from failing to do any cardio for the last two years. At least paralysis is a good excuse? But fragility, I don't think, should be a word to describe me.

11. Funny enough, I made a Facebook post while writing this to figure out what type of gas station was paired with the McDonald's. Don, Dave's Facebook enemy, came up with "McGasoline," which is funny and serendipitous for this story.

12. A WV delicacy. In many ways, this book is my strange ode to WV.

13. It is not lost on me that this is very reminiscent of Jan from *The Office*. Emily's first question is, "Do you think he's going to make you sleep on a tiny cot at the end of the bed?"

14. This was the time of Covid when no one really quite knew what the proper symptoms were, so anything out of the ordinary was cause for concern.

15. Powder and Puff are all white but not albino. Their eyes are brown. We believe this is due to a genetic abnormality. My dad, the first to spot Powder as a fawn, believed that a goat had taken up residence in one of our bushes. He called my mom to come home from work so she could check out the goat and call whomever it belonged to. Does this sound weird to you? Well, welcome to Harrisville, West Virginia, where happenings of this nature make the weekly county paper. When Powder jumped up and stretched, my dad called my mom back to tell her to get home faster. This was no goat but a mythical creature.

16. That's for you, Shelley.

17. Pronounced Care-oh, rhyming with pharaoh.

1. There was also Murphy, a guy I was texting daily. He was super nice, but I became overwhelmed when he sent me a picture of everything I'd ever written (acquired from Amazon) and professed he "did a thing." I panicked because I wanted to tell him my story before a book did, and I never talked to him again. Not my proudest moment, and Murphy, if you're still reading my books, I'm sorry.

2. A version of this section is upcoming as a short story in the *Santa Fe Literary Review* and was recognized at the WV Writers Awards.

3. Okay, there are no big towns around here, so I'm not sure why I make the distinction, but still.

4. Polyfluoroalkyl substances, most often found in Teflon.

5. The microgeneration born 1977-1985, also known as the Oregon Trail Generation.
6. One of those jobs was writing fake reviews of espresso machines and tents on Amazon. I received $3 per 600-word review. If you ever need someone to provide you with multiple synonyms of *camping, stakes, coffee*, or *caffeine*, hit me up.
7. Once, Timmatthew texted me and said, *We out. Karaoke going on. You go to the bathroom and return to find me on stage singing to you.* To this day, Emily and I still laugh about that ridiculous text.
8. See also: limerence.
9. Pronounced *Cunnaw*.
10. Part grandmother, part poor Appalachian, and 100% rock and roll, The Amazing Delores was a Charleston gem who was featured in a documentary series by Jacob Young (most famous for Jesco White's *Dancing Outlaw*) called *Different Drummer*. The Amazing Delores performed all over Charleston in her outrageously sequined outfits. Naturally, Sarah and I are obsessed with her.
11. See Sylvia Plath's "Tulips."
12. We still chat occasionally. He told me he bought my second book. I hope he is well and sending different newds now.

1. The television show, not the titty restaurant where my sister and I showed up early in the morning.
2. Okay, if you remember, there was a point in late 2020 when we all thought you could only get Covid once, and if you had the antigens, you were good to go forever. We all know better now, but back then (and it seems so far away), this was a good sign for me. I didn't have to worry about this guy giving me Covid! He had done his part. He had suffered for all of us.
3. Are you shaved? Do you like anal? Do you hookup?
4. Uncle Mack, if you're reading this, there have been too many to name.
5. One day, I want to get Jeramy tipsy and have him give a Drunk History of Moonville.
6. Although it's not part of the original North Bend tunnels, one of those tunnels is active. Therefore, I substituted Moonville to the quest.
7. If you weren't part of Greek life in college (I wasn't), some fraternity and sorority houses actually come with their own chefs. So fancy.
8. The Flatwoods Monster, obviously.

NOTES

1. It's a lyric from a 90s song by The Presidents of the United States of America, though many Boomers believed I actually received free peaches at the site.
2. I can't help but still call tofu *tubu* to this day.
3. Later research tells me the pronghorn isn't actually a *true* antelope, but the closest thing America has to one. Good enough, I suppose.

1. The tallest person in history for which there is evidence.
2. I lose it and burst into tears after this happened. I heard the techs discussing how they had to send a guy home because they couldn't get his IV in, and I thought this might happen to me. They felt horrible and assured me I wouldn't have to go home until they got this done.
3. I like Liz, though. This does not apply to her.
4. I will say that Idaho is a lawless place. Beautiful but lawless. I drove over the state line once to go to the Moscow, Idaho Wal-Mart, and there was a dog running around with no owner and no leash. Just running around the aisles like he was on some kind of mission from Bigfoot. GET SOME MARSHMALLOWS, DOGGO.
5. I don't write this in a disparaging way, but one of the only nurses who could get my IVs in The Dash's hospital was a former heroin addict who admitted her past life gave her special skills when doing IV stabs in the hospital. She never missed. I commend her.
6. Shoutout to Nuke's Top 5.